A BLESSING
NOT A CURSE

A BLESSING
NOT A CURSE

• • •

A mother-daughter
guide to the
transition from
child to woman

Jane Bennett

SALLY MILNER PUBLISHING

To my mother's mother,

my mother and my daughter

First published in 2002 by
Sally Milner Publishing Pty Ltd
PO Box 2104
Bowral NSW 2576
AUSTRALIA

© Jane Bennett 2002

Design by Anna Warren, Warren Ventures Pty Ltd, Sydney

Illustrations by Rhyll Plant

Edited by Patricia Hoyle

Printed in Australia by McPherson's Printing Group

Cover detail: Marble Sculpture 'Maria', by David Lowe, Queensland

Bennett, Jane.
    Blessing not a curse.

    Bibliography.
    Includes index.
    ISBN 1 86351 300 0.

    1. Menstruation. 2. Menstruation - Psychological aspects.
    3. Menstruation - Social aspects. I. Title. (Series :
    Milner health series).

    612.662

Contents

Acknowledgements

I am amazed and moved when I think of how many people have nourished my book idea with their time, their expertise, their optimism and enthusiasm, their resources and stories, and their love and blessings in order for it to take shape and emerge, whole into the world.

My thanks go to all those who have researched and written on this topic before me, whose material has inspired and made this contribution possible, and especially to Francesca Naish for the years of her invaluable mentoring and awesome example.

I also thank the practitioners and staff at the Jocelyn Centre for Natural Fertility Management and Holistic Medicine for their dedicated and skillful work promoting natural fertility management and healthy menstrual cycles. Similarly the hundreds of health practitioners who studied natural fertility management and preconception health care with us and offer these modalities to their patients with such enthusiasm.

Melinda Smith, Ronnie Moule, Dorothy Douglas, Cheryl Dingle, Daniel Saulwick and Martha Lourey Bird I thank for generously sharing of their time and professional expertise. And also the dedicated librarians of the Castlemaine Library for their help with countless details.

My dear friends Jane Watson, Karen Masman, Alexandra Pope, Toni Pellas, Virginia Louey and Samantha Fairchild I thank for their faith, encouragement and the odd hearty push. For their generous sharing of space, invaluable for the writing process, thank you to Judy

Munro, Elizabeth and Neville Burgess, and David Flanagan and to all my family for the constancy of their support and love.

Thank you to Margaret Bennett, Jeanette Davis, Diana Holden, Catherine Wells, Lynn Dean, Vanita Hayzell, Amber Smith, Rebecca and Chris Schang, Freya McIntosh, Rosie Campbell, Sarah Mitchell, Elizabeth McAlpine, Claire from the beach in Koh Chang, Jane Watson, Jacinta Williams and Jenni Bourke for their menstrual and menarche stories.

I feel very fortunate to have worked with, and want to thank, my publishers Libby Renney and Ian Webster for their imaginative appreciation of a sketchy idea and practical abilities to turn it into reality, my illustrator Rhyll Plant for her great skill and sensitive drawings, and my editor Patricia Hoyle for her respectful, sensitive and skillful editing.

My deep appreciation and love to Kim Lai for his generous support of the writing process, and all the other odd twists of life.

And thank you for giving reality to these thoughts by picking up *A Blessing Not a Curse* and contemplating the ideas and information. I hope you find it stimulating, useful and at least a bit challenging. May you and your daughter experience a joyful exploration of your natural rhythms and cyclical time, and know menstrual wellness and menstrual blessings.

Honouring menstruation

S usan's mother had told her that women had periods in order to have babies and that some day she would begin to bleed. Her period began one day when she was thirteen. Susan changed her underwear, got a pad and belt from the bathroom cupboard and put it on as her mother had shown her. Then she went to her room, closed the door and sat on her bed. She felt as though her life was over. She couldn't even cry. Except for perhaps when she had babies, she thought she was going to bleed until she was old.

Recently, a girl was brought into the emergency department of a regional hospital extremely distressed and unable to tell her mother what was the matter. It took staff and her mother an hour to calm her down enough to discover her period had begun. She and her family were active in a local church with a fire and brimstone approach to sin and retribution. Knowing nothing about menstruation, she thought her sins and bad thoughts had manifested in this bleeding from the most shameful part of her body, that she would slowly bleed to death.

One day a man heard a story about a girl who had no knowledge of menstruation when she first started to bleed. She felt utterly devastated and alone. Having no-one she felt she could confide in, she committed suicide. When he heard this story the man was profoundly moved and vowed that no-one should be that alone again. He went on to found a free anonymous 24-hour telephone counselling service.

Views of menstruation as a sickness, as something to endure that we would be better off without, an embarrassment and a curse, are very common. Reflected in the early menstrual experiences of many women, this is true now and across time, and in many cultures. These attitudes are still preserved by taboos and social institutions, as well as in subtle inter-personal and inter-generational ways.

Shame about menstruation has come from many sources. In Western society, loss of a natural perception of menstruation began generations ago when women whose mothers (perhaps those who burned as witches) broke the tradition of teaching, preparing, and welcoming their daughters into this fundamental aspect of being a woman. Millions of young women over countless generations lost their inheritance of the miraculous body and instead feared that they were dying, diseased, or were being punished by God. A woman's time of heightened sensation, intuition, feeling, and creativity was turned into a time of humiliation shame and punishment.

> When I started to bleed for the first time I didn't know anything about menstruation or cycles or women's fertility. I thought I was hemorrhaging and would soon die. I was very frightened, but strangely calm at the same time. Of course it proved to be the curse. (Julia)

YOUR ROLE AS PARENT

Menarche (first menstruation) is a time of profound change, the beginning of 35 to 40 years of fertility, cycling and menstruation. It's a vulnerable time, especially for girls unprepared or ill-prepared, and the experiences of this time can impact negatively or positively, on later menstrual experiences.

With overtones of 'curse' ruling this primary and universal feminine experience, we're right to be concerned. But there is much you can do! Research has shown that a mother's influence is considerable, even primary, in her daughter's experience of menarche and menstruation (Mahr 1987, Patton, Hibbert and Cartlin 1996).

If you honour and celebrate menstruation and the menstrual cycle, or at the least 'normalise' it, you will promote a deep level of self-acceptance in your daughter (and yourself); a self-acceptance that many women strive for but have difficulty achieving. To do this you need to become aware of your cultural heritage regarding 'the curse', which permeates religion, science, medicine, media and literature, commerce and advertising, as well as your own family views and values. If you're familiar with the changes of the menstrual cycle, and your own cycle, it will be easier to answer your daughter's questions before and after menarche.

While the whole complexity of cultural 'discomforts', if not full-'blooded' taboos around menstruating women, aren't simple to redress, positive (real) and open information offers most to girls of this age, and needs to be openly and widely available on an ongoing basis. When you offer her knowledge, she will come back to you again and again as her understanding and experience changes and grows. You can consult books or a specialist for information and/or therapy, and your attitude of 'let's go and find out' will support a positive overall approach towards menstruation that your daughter will imbibe from you.

Girls who have a positive experience of menarche and their ongoing menstrual cycle are able to naturally grow into the in-drawing centredness, the confidence, the groundedness, that conscious, positive and healthy menstruating can offer. Menstruation is an aspect of their blossoming sexuality — an inward time to be with themselves, a time to explore their changes and start to get to know the fertile and infertile times of their menstrual cycle, *before* they begin a sexual relationship.

Although menstruation is, practically speaking, 'women's business', I believe understanding, knowledge and experiences of menstruation should not be kept from men or boys. In all our relationships, whether as husband and wife, father and daughter, brother and sister, friend and friend, colleague and colleague, we can all benefit by understanding each other better, including sharing experiences and knowledge about menstruation.

Generally men and boys learn their attitudes about menstruation from the women in their life, usually at home from their mother, and sometimes father, from one generation to the next. Silence and evasion teach as much as any other method. Jokes and accusations of being 'on the rag' and such like are offensive, and may occur at school, in the office, and even in homes — these are not attitudes born of openness, information and respect. It's up to women to help men and boys understand menstruation better by talking about it, by understanding it better ourselves, by being open and helping the men in our lives overcome any fear or misunderstanding they may have about the female cycle.

> At my school the boys would often pinch girls on the bum to see if they were wearing pads. If they were then this would lead to lots of teasing. Apart from a hurried lesson one afternoon in first year there was not much discussion about periods — there certainly were some pretty negative views going around, and the situation was mortifying for the girls. Hard to believe this was only fifteen years ago — hope things have changed there since.
> (Catherine)

There is a school of thought that blames patriarchy for prevailing attitudes and experiences of menstruation. Although many of the forces that created and perpetuated the 'curse' were male dominated, or exclusively male, institutions, in our modern world blaming men for 'the curse' only perpetuates powerlessness (not to be confused with consideration of causes and growing awareness). To a great extent it's women who now have the power to examine and change prevailing attitudes.

> One day after school I was walking with some friends in a local shopping centre. Nearby were some boys from a higher form at our school. One came up to me and whispered 'I think your period has come', simply and kindly. It had come and I didn't know. I had a big

stain on the back of my tunic. My friends either hadn't seen or
didn't want to say. I really had a crush on that boy for a while.
(Lynn)

So, although (for simplicity of style and because the majority of
readers will be mothers) I refer to readers as mothers, I am aware that
fathers and other caregivers will be interested in this subject. I deeply
honour your interest and valuable influence in the lives of daughters
and girls and ask you to include yourself as 'universal mothers' when
reading this book. The special and specific role of fathers, and other
significant males, is also addressed in Part 3, Rite of Passage.

YOUR GUIDE

A Blessing Not a Curse will guide you in the importance and meaning
of preparing girls well for menarche and the vital role you play as her
mother, father or carer.

Part 1 Our Cycling Bodies, lays the groundwork for understanding
the psychological and physical nature of cycles and menstruation. We
then explore in Part 2 Blessing or Curse? the cultural and historical
legacies, and medical views of 'the curse', and their impact on the
experiences of girls and women individually and collectively. An
alternative view of menstruation as a blessing follows — the
incredible, but largely unexplored or forgotten, physio-psycho-
spiritual potential of the menstrual cycle beyond the miracle of
reproduction and beyond healthy attitudes to healthy cycles.

In Part 3 Rite of Passage you'll find questions designed to help you
remember and unfold your own experiences, followed by practical
advice on how to talk to your daughter and make menarche a time of
celebration. There are also questions for men.

In Part 4, Problem Periods and Part 5, Learning to Ride the
Menstrual Cycle, you will learn how to guide your daughter with self-
help methods for healthy cycles and when to seek what kind of
professional help.

A Blessing Not a Curse will help you unfold your experience of menstruation and the menstrual cycle to discover the riches hidden within your own experiences. Through this process, and the practical guidelines offered throughout the book, you'll be empowered to offer your daughter a graceful entry into, and positive unfolding of, her menstrual journey as she blossoms gorgeously into a strong and centred woman.

Part 1

Our cycling bodies

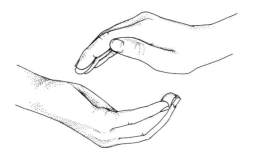

1. A natural rhythm

A natural bodily rhythm, our cycle continues whether we're conscious of it or not. Sometimes the premenstrum nudges into our awareness through bloating, irritability or lethargy. Often we're only aware of the bleeding, and any cramping or pain that accompanies it — our period has arrived. Yet, like the seasons, night and day, the circling planets and galaxies, or simply breathing in and out, the cycle continues.

For all women, and for at least half of their lives, menstruation is the most obvious sign of the ongoing hormonal cycle with emotional and psychic changes manifesting in complex and powerful ways. Each menstrual cycle has similarities, while at the same time each one is different — the variables are infinite.

We are always in flux, constant in our changes, steady in our pulsing rhythms. At all stages of the cycle, many subtle (and some not so subtle) changes are taking place within our bodies and psyche. Even without deliberately setting out to track her cycle, by the nature of its rhythms, a woman will be aware of changes, even though many are subliminal. This tunes her in to her body and herself. Women's experience of this is varied, but like the joy a gardener has in the seasons of his garden, or a yogini in the rhythms of her breath, a woman can derive great joy in the rhythm of her cycling body. And many do.

Although individual women's experiences vary, research has shown that women are, on average, significantly more aware of their bodies than men and relate more flexibly to their bodies. The menstrual cycle is probably what gives them this advantage. A woman experiences the rhythmic and profound changes in her body (as well as the even more profound changes of pregnancy, birth and lactation for those who become mothers), as her menstrual cycle waxes and wanes. For men there is no comparable experience. Most men are probably happy enough with this, although some cultures have bloodletting menstrual rituals for men, including a number of Australian aboriginal tribes, the Caraja and Javahe tribes of the Amazon River and the Wogeo from an island off the coast of New Guinea. Blood sports and war have often been attributed to 'menstrual envy'.

MENSTRUATION AND THE MOON

The word *menstruation* comes from the Latin and Greek words for *month* and *moon*. Mensis means moon in Latin, and many other languages have words for menstruation that correspond to their words for moon. Not surprisingly the average length of the menstrual cycle is the same as the lunar cycle at approximately 29.5 days. The moon is also a cycling body and our personal relationship to the lunar cycle is a form of biorhythm that starts at birth, becomes effective at puberty, and continues to influence our fertility throughout our fertile life (Naish 1993). As the moon cycles graciously around our planet it becomes a metaphor and our patroness — we too can learn to cycle graciously.

Throughout history and cultures women's cycles have been acknowledged as connected with the moon. Native American women traditionally prayed to the moon to help them with irregular cycles. Bahloo, an important Australian Aboriginal moon deity, helped to create girl babies. The Maori of New Zealand called menstruation mata marama, moon sickness, and believed a girl's first period to be caused by the moon seducing her while she slept. In parts of India and the Torres Strait Islands one word is used for both moon and menstrual blood.

In the 1940s and 50s there was growing evidence of the moon's influence upon the body rhythms and fertility of a wide range of animals and plants. The metabolic and sexual activity of many animals ranging from oysters and worms to monkeys and cows and plant life (including potatoes, carrots and seaweed) have been found to vary with specific phases of the moon *even when removed from the influence of tides and moonlight* (Naish, 1993). There is also evidence of changes in human psycho-sexual response relative to the phases of the moon.

Studies have shown that peak rates for conception are around the full moon, indicating that this is the peak time for ovulation, ovulation and conception rates being significantly less at the new moon, when more women are menstruating (Northrup, 1994).

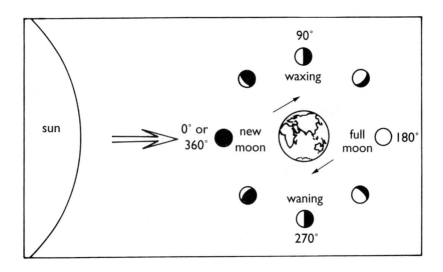

The lunar cycle

Dr Eugine Jonas discovered (or perhaps more accurately, rediscovered) in the 1960s another powerful proof of our intimate connection with the moon. He found that along with her hormonal cycle a woman has a second cycle that relates to the lunar cycle. Dr Jonas found that every time the angle between the sun and moon, relative to the earth, is the same as at a woman's birth (which happens once every 29.5 days approximately) she has the capacity to spontaneously ovulate, irrespective of where she is in her hormonal cycle. This finding elaborated upon the work of researchers like Masters and Johnson who discovered that women do have the capacity to spontaneously ovulate at other times than their hormonal ovulation (Naish, 1993).

WHY DO WE MENSTRUATE?

Many mammals reproduce without menstruating. So menstruation is not just about perpetuating the species. Although it's not certain why humans menstruate, there are many interesting theories and new theories continue to emerge.

A current favourite is the energy efficient theory of menstruation, proposed by Beverly Strassman from the University of Michigan, which relates to the energetic needs of the human brain. The placenta must be large and rich to support the growth of the foetal brain and the placenta feeds on blood. Pound for pound brain tissue is ten times more expensive to maintain than any other tissue of the human body. To support a potential embryo and placenta, the endometrium right after ovulation needs to be thick, rich and metabolically dynamic, secreting hormones, proteins, fats, sugars, nucleic acids. So the endometrium is energetically dear, using seven times the oxygen used when the endometrium is at its thinnest. The endometrial secretions influence the entire body from brain to bowel, requiring higher metabolism and more calories.

If there is no embryo to nourish, this rich lining becomes a burden to maintain. Strassman estimates that in four months of cycling a woman saves an amount of energy equal to six days worth of food over what she would have needed to maintain a perpetually active endometrium. It is therefore cheaper, energetically, to build up a rich endometrial lining and to shed it than to maintain it in perpetually readiness (Strassmann 1996 in Angier1999).

2. The menstrual cycle

THE INTERPLAY OF HORMONES

The most amazing messengers of rhythm and balance and response, hormones regulate all our bodily functions as well as our emotional and psychic states. In turn, our environment and emotional state influence our hormonal balance.

Powerful chemical substances, in minuscule quantities, hormones are measured in laboratories in billionths or trillionths of a gram. To get one teaspoon of estradiol (the predominant oestrogen) we would need the blood of a quarter of a million cycling women. In comparison, the blood supply of any one of us would contain at least one teaspoon of sugar and several teaspoons of salt (Angier, 1999). Even in these exquisitely small quantities a little too much (or too little) oestrogen, for example, will throw us right off balance. And not just our menstrual cycle, but many other physiological functions like heart rate and metabolism as well.

The endocrine glands are the major hormone producers and the main glands that produce the hormones which regulate the menstrual cycle are the hypothalamus, the pituitary and the ovary. The hypothalamus is at the base of the brain and controls body functions. In it is a specialised portion called the menstrual clock which is responsible for the periodic time of the menstrual cycle. Our hormones swirl through our system in an exquisite dance — as one hormone level diminishes this triggers the release of another, choreographing the menstrual ballet month after month.

While we're not consciously aware of the subtleties of the

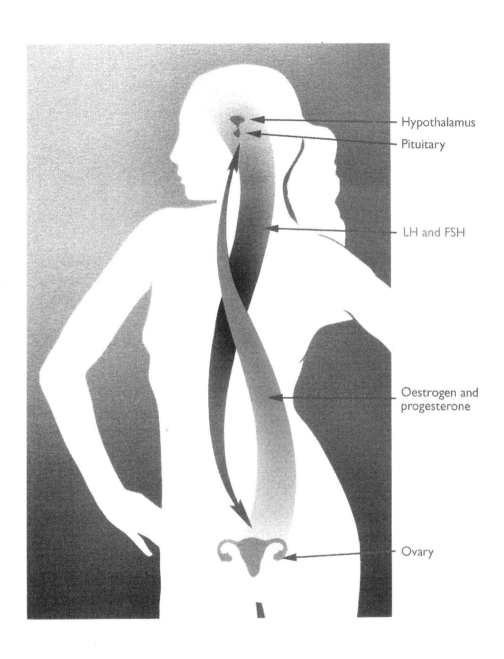

Hypothalamus

Pituitary

LH and FSH

Oestrogen and
progesterone

Ovary

Hypothalamus, pituitary and ovary

menstrual cycle, our cycle is sensitive to us, intimately in contact with our brain and body. The triggers of the first half of the cycle are especially sensitive to factors such as stress, ill health, long distance travel and emotions, which can all influence an early or delayed hormonal release. While cycles may vary in length from three weeks to forty days, the *average* cycle is twenty-nine and a half days. Almost all the variation is between menstruation and ovulation — once ovulation has occurred the remainder of the cycle tends to be close to fourteen days, give or take a day or two.

THE PERIOD BEGINS

Menstruation, or bleeding, is the most universally recognised experience of the cycle, with the first day of menstruation becoming 'day one'. While in this book I present the menstrual cycle in a linear way to explain it more clearly, hold onto the concept that the menstrual cycle is *circular, round and womanly*, not linear.

Just before menstruation, the endometrium (the lining of the womb) has reached its maximum thickness of about 8 millimetres. The spiral corkscrew arteries of the endometrium constrict sharply, stopping blood flow, then open again suddenly, releasing blood that pools beneath the endometrium causing the lining to swell and burst. Uterine contractions help the menstrual blood on its way out through the cervix and down the vagina. Menstruation begins.

Menstruation is when the menstrual blood flows rather than just 'spotting', which may occur for a day or two before menstruation begins. The average period lasts for between three to five days.

Menstrual blood itself is much more than just blood. The average period is two or three tablespoons in volume, half of it blood and the other half the remains of the uterine lining, egg cells, oestrogenic hormones, lecithins, arsenic compounds and rich concentrations of essential minerals, such as iron and phosphorous, along with vaginal and cervical secretions. Menstrual blood doesn't clot (although tissues in it may be clotty) as the blood itself has very few platelets and

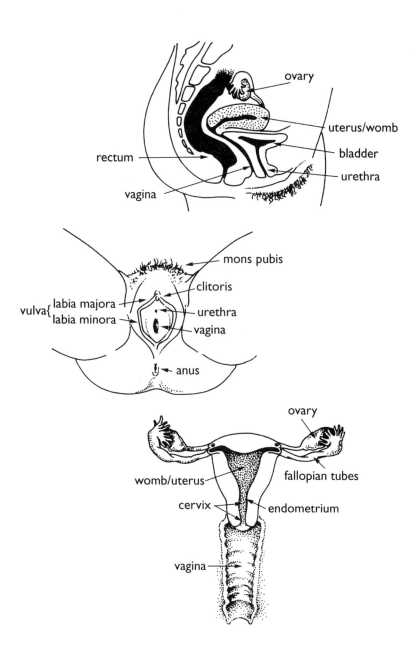

Cross section of female reproductive organs

therefore does not form the necessary interlocking coagulatory mesh for clotting (Angier,1999).

Over a million menstruating women

In Australia there are about 5,500,000 cycling girls and women, and over one million women menstruating at any one time. With each average cycle approximately 275,000 litres of menstrual blood flows in Australia, or 9,322 litres per day. Worldwide about 275 million women are menstruating at any one time (approximately the entire population of the United States) amounting to about 7.4 million litres of menstrual blood a day or 2.7 billion litres a year.

Each menstruation produces between 30 to 60 millilitres of blood and tissue, but may vary from 10 millilitres to 300 millilitres in individual women. The average woman with the average menstrual volume will release about 20 litres of menstrual blood in her lifetime, and will spend an average of six and a half years menstruating (Trickey,1998, Van De Graaff,1989, Australian Bureau of Statistics,2001).

THE FOLLICLE MATURES

With very few, if any, hormones being released from the ovaries at menstruation, the hypothalamus is signaled to produce gonadatrophin releasing hormone (GnRH) which in turn stimulates the pituitary gland just below it to produce lutenising hormone (LH) and follicle stimulating hormone (FSH). The LH and FSH stimulate the ovary to release progesterone and oestrogen, which is recognised by the hypothalamus and reminds it to produce GnRH. And around the signals go in a hormonal feedback loop. The LH and FSH signals to the ovaries to stimulate the expansion and ripening of around 10 to 20 follicles, each containing an immature egg.

This phase of the cycle, known as the ovarian follicular phase, begins on day one of the cycle (the day menstruation begins) and lasts until ovulation. While the follicles are developing they are producing more and more oestrogen which stimulates the endometrium, the cells lining the uterus, to grow and proliferate. The endometrium thickens from about 1 millimetre at the end of the period to about 6 millimetres by ovulation. This uterine proliferative phase starts on between day three and day six of the cycle and continues until ovulation, at around day fourteen.

As levels of oestrogen change through the cycle they cause the cervix to soften and rise and its opening, the os, to widen. The mucus produced in the crypts also changes in quantity and quality from alkaline and very scant to becoming more profuse, acid and 'fertile'.

Three or four days before ovulation one of the ripening follicle-eggs is chosen to reach full maturity and ovulate (occasionally more are chosen and if fertilised you get fraternal twins, triplets and so on). Those not chosen diminish. The chosen follicle continues to develop — the egg within it matures and its chromosomes are sorted through a process called meiosis (Angier 1999).

By the time it's ready to ovulate, the follicle containing the mature egg is so engorged that it measures up to 1 centimetre across. The delicate ends of the fallopian tubes, with their sensitive sea-creature-like waving fingers (fimbriae) have been brushing over the ovary feeling for signs of where the follicle will burst, to be ready for the precious egg as it is released. The flexible fallopian tubes can even reach over to the opposite ovary if the tube closest to it is somehow incapacitated (for example by endometriosis adhesions).

Our menstrual abundance

At seven months in-utero a female foetus has the most eggs that she will ever have — five million. By the time she is born, a baby girl has one million eggs, and by the time she reaches puberty 350,000 remain — they're all gone by menopause. At puberty, as eggs begin to mature and

---

are released from one ovary then another, the ovulation-menstruation cycle begins.

With the average menarche (onset of periods) at around 12 years old and the average menopause at around 50, the average woman cycles and menstruates for approximately 38 years. The average length of a cycle is 29.5 days, giving about 12.25 cycles a year. If we take out 2.5 years for the average number of pregnancies and the post-natal anovulatory period, we then have 35.5 years of cycling, times 12.25 cycles per year which means the average woman will have 435 cycles in her lifetime. Our own number of cycles could be anywhere between 360 and 500.

THE EGG IS RELEASED

The day of ovulation is the beginning of the ovarian luteal phase, named after the corpus luteum, which lasts about fourteen days until the next period begins. The final signal for ovulation comes from the pituitary gland in the form of a great whoosh of luteinizing hormone (LH) and follicle stimulating hormone (FSH) which stimulates the follicle to burst and release the egg. The tiny hair-like projections on the fimbriae at the end of the waiting fallopian tubes all wave in synchrony and create a current which draws the egg into and along the tube.

Meanwhile, back at the ovary, the ruptured follicle lives on to become a temporary gland producing hormones to nourish its released egg. The hormones progesterone (more) and oestrogen (less) course into the bloodstream and cause the uterine lining to grow. They also stimulate the breasts, producing some swelling or tenderness, as well as influence every other organ in the woman's body. The luteal phase corresponds to the secretary phase of the endometrium (see chart: hormone levels and their effects through the menstrual cycle on page 27). Progesterone and oestrogen also cause the endometrium to build up a glycogen-rich tissue, a suitable bed for a fertilised egg should one arrive. In addition, progesterone causes the

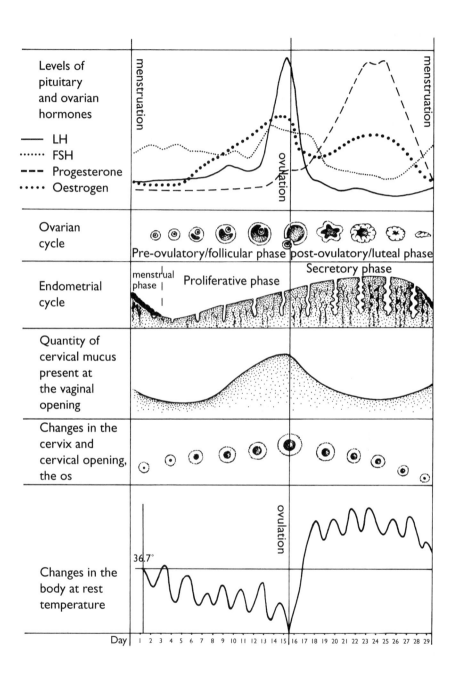

Hormone levels and their effects through the menstrual cycle

body-at-rest temperature to rise, the cervical mucus to lessen and thicken, the lining of the womb to thicken more and be fully supplied with nutrients, and the ovary to stop releasing eggs.

The follicle cells fill up with cholesterol and turn soft and yellow, forming the corpus luteum, meaning 'yellow body'. The lifespan of the corpus luteum is about 12 to 16 days (unless conception occurs when it lives on to support the pregnancy). This doesn't vary much from woman to woman or cycle to cycle. When its usefulness is over, macrophages (the immune system cells) clean up the used cells of the corpus luteum, and fibrous tissue forms. The corpus luteum becomes the corpus albicans (the white body) — another small white scar on the ovarian wall.

As the corpus luteum dies and ovarian hormonal secretion falls, the menstrual phase of the endometrial cycle is triggered and the cycle begins once again.

Our ever changing body

During the menstrual cycle there are measurable changes in *most* body factors including:

- Sex hormone levels in blood and urine
- Buccal, rectal and vaginal temperatures
- Basal metabolism
- Blood sugar
- Endometrial glycogen
- Water retention
- Body weight
- Pulmonary vital capacity
- Alveolar CO_2 concentrations
- Arterial oxygen pressure
- Blood acidity
- Serum bicarbonate
- Heart rate

- Erythrocyte sedimentation rate
- Differential blood leucocyte counts
- Platelet counts
- Serum protein
- Vitamins A, C and E concentrations
- Bile pigments
- Blood adrenalin
- Urine volume
- Thyroid and adrenal function
- Electric skin resistance
- Pupillary size
- Psychic activities
- Pain threshold
- Skin colour and permeability
- Breast changes
- Composition of cervical mucous secretion and citric acid content
- Viscosity and gravity of urine
- Work performance
- Electro-encephalogram readings (brain waves)
- Olfactory, visual and auditory acuity
- The ability to walk the tightrope!
- Size, position and colour of the cervix

(Van De Graaff 1989 and Naish 1993)

THE PSYCHOLOGICAL CYCLE

Many psychological, emotional and spiritual changes accompany the all-encompassing physical changes of the menstrual cycle. In her book *Women's Bodies, Women's Wisdom*, Christiane Northrup reports on research and her clinical findings that the first half of the cycle (the luteal phase between menstruation and ovulation) is a good time for ideas, creativity and beginning new projects. Ovulation represents mental and emotional creativity at its peak and the luteal phase (between ovulation and menstruation) is an evaluative and reflective time, a time when we're preparing to give birth to something from deep within. At menstruation we experience a physical and psychological release — it is a cleansing and simplifying time (Northrup 1994).

As an example of the psychological impact of the menstrual cycle, a study of 84 female undergraduates, ranging from 17 to 27 years found a significant relationship between personal space and the menstrual cycle — the amount of personal space (or the personal space zone) required tended to be larger during the menstrual flow than during the approximate middle of the cycle (Sanders 1978).

Many other variables of psychological state are found to cycle with the menstrual cycle, some common to many women and others more specific to individual women. To become more familiar with your own you can chart your cycle and include psychological variables in your charting (see Appendix 1).

I think that what's happening to me is so wonderful, and I don't just mean the changes taking place on the outside of my body, but also those on the inside. I never discuss myself or any of these things with others, which is why I have to talk about them to myself. Whenever I get my period (and that's only been three times), I have the feeling that in spite of all the pain, discomfort and mess, I'm carrying around a sweet secret. So even though it's a nuisance, in a certain way I'm always looking forward to the time when I'll feel that secret inside me once again. (Anne Frank)
(Frank, 1991,pg 158-9)

Part 2

Blessing
or
Curse?

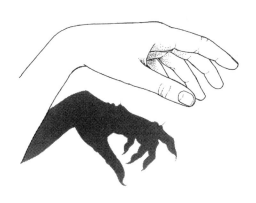

1. Curse

There are few themes recurring so often throughout the modern world and through history as the idea that menstruation is shameful and a threat to all concerned. Defined as a 'curse', traditionally menstruation was thought to give women extra powers to curse (and sometimes to bless). To curse means '… to utter against (persons or things) words which consign them to evil; to damn; to anathematise; to afflict with such evils as indicate divine wrath or a malignant fate; the evil inflicted in response to an imprecation, or in the way of retribution; a thing which blights or blasts … slang for menstruation.' (Oxford English Dictionary).

The pervasive view of menstruation still has little to do with menstruation as a healthy, natural aspect of the menstrual cycle, fertility, sexuality, creativity and inspiration. I've even heard women who work in women's health (and so have women's wellbeing at heart) express negative views on menstruation. These are public women and role models. Women who should know better. There is a collective shadow over menstruation and menstruating women — we unconsciously negate or deny menstruation, accepting it as a bad thing. A curse.

In February 1986 I was 15 and on a two week school trip to Russia with a small group to practise our Russian and soak up some Russian culture. We were on an overnight train from Kiev to Moscow and I was sharing a sleeper cabin with my best friend, Robyn. I woke up in the morning with blood on the sheets and, as a way of letting her know my period had come, I said to Robyn, 'I hate being a woman today'. She knew exactly what I meant. I looked out the window, it was light by then, we were moving slowly through a forest of cypress and pine hung heavy with snow. Snow was thick on the ground and on the tracks. It was very beautiful. Later that day, Robyn started to bleed too, and said to me, 'I hate being a woman today too'. It was too embarrassing to say period, although we often called it 'the curse'. Everyone did. (Catherine)

THE SHADOW

The 'shadow' was described by psychologist Carl Jung as our own dark side, characterised by what we judge as 'inferior, uncivilised or animal' qualities which the ego wishes to hide from others as our 'shadow'. Our individual shadow is always the same sex as ourselves. The shadow is something no person consciously wants to be — wild and unsocialised. Yet when we become 'civilised' it's at the expense of spontaneity, creativity, strong emotions, deep insights, the wisdom of instinctual nature, a wisdom that may be more profound than that which any learning or culture can provide. A shadowless life becomes shallow and spiritless, and may result in a collapse into helplessness and ill-health.

But the shadow is persistent and won't easily be suppressed. Through integration, when the ego and shadow work in close harmony, the shadow is brought to consciousness — we feel full of life and vigour, our consciousness is expanded and we feel more physically and mentally vital, alive and vigorous.

The forces of a collective shadow are evident in any mass movement, trend, or gathering, or by the denial and negative attitudes expressed towards it. The writer D.H. Lawrence described the shadow as 'a conflict between the white mental consciousness and the deep red 'blood self''. When a shadow is stringently repressed by society, or when it has inadequate outlets, there is often disaster. Writing in 1918 at the end of World War I, Jung observed that the 'animal in us only becomes more beast-like' when it is repressed.

Even the number thirteen has long been endowed with shadowy qualities, and pops up in stories, folk-law and modern city hotels (which often don't have a 13th floor)! The solar year is divided into twelve solar months, while the lunar year and the menstrual year has months of approximately 29.5 days (sometimes incorrectly said to be 28 days) —more than twelve in a year. Approximately every third year will have thirteen full moons, and a woman with an average and regular cycle will have thirteen menstrual periods.

Both dangerous and powerful, the number thirteen itself came to be seen as a shadow — the number that represents menstruation, the moon, the curse and women's connection with it. Sleeping Beauty's father, in his denial of his daughter's inevitable menstruation, fertility and sexuality, did not invite the thirteenth wise woman to bless her at her christening. To 'forget' the thirteenth wise woman is to deny her blessing of menstruation and as menstruation *will come* it will then come as a curse.

On shadows, perhaps Clarrisa Pinkola Estes has the final wise word: 'The shadow also, however, can contain the divine, the luscious, beautiful, and powerful aspects of personhood. For women especially, the shadow almost always contains very fine aspects of being that are forbidden or given little support by her culture. At the bottom of the well in the psyches of too many women lies the visionary creator, the astute truth-teller, the far-seer, the one who can speak well of herself without denigration, who can face herself without cringing, who works to perfect her craft. The positive impulses in shadow for women of our culture most often revolve around permission for the creation of a hand-made life.' (Estes 1992, p. 236).

THE LEGACY OF THE WITCH HUNTS

The witch hunts of the Middle Ages are a classic example of unintegrated shadow. In Christianity the feminine traditionally became equated with either the Virgin Mary or with the wicked temptress Eve. Everything of the feminine which was not the impossibly virginal, pure, white and unearthly Mary, became the shadow — the natural cycles of women, the blood, the connection with natural rhythms, the knowing by women of the earth and moon cycles, the natural wildness, the powerful bringing forth of new life. All that was not Mary became 'witch' and was persecuted.

In 1484 Pope Innocent VIII authorised two Dominican priests to write the *Malleus Maleficarum*, a handbook defining what witches did, how they were alleged to do it, and how to sentence them. Over three centuries it's estimated that nine million people (one hundred women to every man) were sentenced and murdered as witches by the church. Burning witches at the stake was designed specifically to kill without spilling blood. The power and danger was believed to be in the witch's blood and the *Malleus Maleficarum* stated 'Thou shalt not spill a witches blood'.

The evils of witches were described in the *Malleus Maleficarum* in the same way the Western Christian Church of the day described the evils of menstruating women. The church identified women with sin and a satanised sexuality, promoting a world and church in which only men and a male trinity had power. If a woman died in childbirth, or while menstruating, her family was not allowed to bury her in consecrated ground.

A fourteenth century Christian church edict said 'If a women dare to cure without having studied, she is a witch and must die'. 'Study' was church defined and available only to men. This was also a class issue as the poor couldn't afford the fees of male physicians and were succoured mostly by women who had gained some skill in healing. Nature was the teacher of these women, not scripture, and they were reviled and persecuted.

The basis of witch persecution is the profound misunderstanding, mistrust and fear of how a woman's power grows with the moon and comes and goes with it, and how through their bodies and, in particular, through their reproductive organs, women are felt to have peculiar and privileged access to medicine of a kind dangerously independent of male control. Descriptions of witches read like descriptions of PMS, menstrual taboos and curses.

Given the magnitude of the witch burning and the suppression of women we can only speculate what was lost to the Western world of the natural crafts of women — healing, herbs, midwifery, dowsing, dream-study, hypnotism, sexual fulfilment, all empowered and underscored by a proper knowledge and understanding of the menstrual and lunar cycles.

The witch remains a shadowy image in our society, mostly in fairy tales, but still that of the feminine — dark and wild with secret powers. She is not ruled by the dominant male culture, but obeys deeper, earthier and more universal rhythms and laws. Perhaps it's this archetype we most embody premenstrually and menstrually when we're at our best, most ourselves, most in touch, intuitive, inspired, creative, seeking to redress imbalances, drawing our power from within and less from without. It's also when we're at our worst, irritable, in pain, not ourselves, even violent, as we try to sustain our own or our culture's linear, non-cyclical mode. Perhaps this is why seclusion is good at this time as it supports our tuning-in at this naturally less worldly, more soulful time.

A CROSS CULTURAL CURSE

The power and the danger, the positive and the negative, the blessing and the curse, are inextricably linked together in a complex web. Common features across cultures are seclusion, taboo, fasting, physical restriction and sometimes, even abuse.

In some cultures women are secluded on their own, and in others in a women's menstrual hut, or tent. The seclusion in some cultures is a desire to isolate the polluting or cursing influence, and in others it's seen as a time for women to be separate from the world of every day concerns, to contain and focus the internal powers of this time in the cycle. Although the menstrual hut can be seen as a place of power or pollution, menstruation always confers a different status, usually with negative connotations that evoke shame along with implications of power and potency.

In Ancient Persia menstruation was considered acceptable only when it lasted no more than four days. During this time, women were isolated in special rooms. After four days, if a woman continued to bleed, she received one hundred lashes and was returned to isolation for another five days. If she continued to menstruate after this time she received a further four hundred lashes as it was believed that she was possessed by a bad spirit, and a 'purification' in the form of whip-lashing was thought to be the cure.

When an Andaman Island girl tells her parents her first blood has come they weep for her, in shame. The girl bathes, then must go into isolation for three days, usually in a specially constructed hut. There she must sit quite still — for the first twenty-four hours she is stripped of all her ornaments and is tied up with cords. She is given a backrest but must not lie down, go to sleep or speak. Her seclusion goes on with less severity for three days. Every day she must wash herself clean of the impurities of menstruation, bathing in the sea for a long time. She then goes back to normal life, but is still expected to bathe every day until her next menstruation.

While Indian village girls are often celebrated with gifts, song and dance at their menarche, there are many taboos relating to where menstruating women may and may not go and what they can do because of the potential harm they may cause. Tantric practitioners in India prize menstrual blood as a powerful substance, all the more from untouchable women, whereas in the general society it's thought the most polluting substance of all.

A menstruating woman is seen by Hindus as impure and are treated like an untouchable, the lowest order of the Hindu caste system. Hindus also believe that a menstruating woman is under the moon's influence and should be treated with respect (as in distance) and care. The Hindu *The Code of Manu* states that a menstruating woman shall be put apart for three days — she is not to look upon anyone until the fourth day when she bathes. Orthodox Hindus are particularly concerned about the touch or glance of a menstruating woman, which is said to spoil food and curdle milk. Not supposed to bathe until after she has finished menstruating the woman then washes thoroughly to become completely purified and renewed.

Chinese tradition speaks poetically of menstruation as the Red Flood, Peach-flower Flow, or the Red Snow. In ancient China it was customary for a woman to separate herself from normal worldly activities during this time — she was not supposed to cook or take part in any family duties or religious rites, and her forehead was generally marked with a red spot to indicate her condition.

When a Muslim woman's period arrives she traditionally recites the Kalima, an article of faith. This ritual marks the beginning of her period of pollution which bars her from fasting, reciting daily prayers or touching the Holy Koran. Within the Islamic holy book the scriptures say that women are subordinate to men because of menstruation.

The traditional Judeo-Christian teachings are that menstruation is polluting and a menstruating women needs to be separate for seven days, as anything she touches, or anyone who touches her, will be unclean. Orthodox Jews require that on the seventh day after menstruation ceases, the polluted woman has a mikvah, a ritual bath, to cleanse her.

The Christian Bible (Leviticus 15:19-33) describes, for fourteen verses and in great detail, the forms of a menstruating woman's uncleanliness and the means by which one can purify oneself after touching her or her things, or eating any food she may have prepared. 'And if a woman have an issue, and her issue in her flesh be blood, she shall be put apart seven days: and whosoever toucheth her shall be unclean until the even...' Leviticus was quoted as the ultimate authority by Senator Ervin in a US Senate session as the reason for not ratifying the Equal Rights Amendment as recently as 1972.

One afternoon our sports teacher, Miss Pritchard, spent a double lesson telling us about periods, the menstrual cycle, sex, conception, relationships, and so on. She was great; really comfortable and she answered all our questions. It was just as well as my period arrived that very evening, for the first time. Mum had never said anything about it. When I told her, she just said 'Oh', and then we went out to buy supplies for me. She was a very devout Anglican, and I think for her periods just weren't nice, to have or to talk about. Even when I had to stay home from school for a day almost every period, from fainting and pain, we never spoke about 'it' directly. (Claire)

A MEDIA CURSE

Despite the large numbers of women menstruating and the amount of time women spend menstruating, menstruation is grossly under-represented, as well as misrepresented, in media and literature.

Advertisements for 'sanitary products' are a fascinating window into social views and resulting legislation about what can and can't be said and seen. In the United States the word 'period' was allowed for the first time on ABC and NBC for Tambrands advertising in 1985. Both networks received written and phoned-in complaints.

Stringent conditions still exist in England including no unwrapped towels or tampons, no suggestion of social insecurity, and 'offensive' words such as 'odour' and 'leakage' are banned. Menstrual products are usually advertised heavily disguised by soft lighting and flowing pastel silks. Many advertising campaigns have laboured to conceal their product in direct contrast to the usual maximum exposure of advertising. Lil-lets advertising has a ball-and-chain theme, reinforcing the idea of menstruation as restriction, even punishment for being a woman.

In Australia menstrual products were banned from being advertised on television, even euphemistically, until 1972. Now even unwrapped products are acceptable, but in some ads a curious blue liquid is poured onto pads to show how it disappears into the nether regions of the product. Such products assume, and sell to the assumption, that women don't want to see their menstrual blood.

The universal use of the words 'sanitary' and 'hygiene' in relation to menstrual products promotes the view that menstrual blood is unclean and unhygienic. In the late 1990s an advertisement appeared in Australia in which a menstrual pad was used by a woman to mop up the spilt blood of her just murdered victim, demonstrating the pad's powers of absorption. This is the first time 'real-red' blood has ever been used in menstrual product advertising. We live in a society willing to accept the numbing frequency of witnessing the blood of violence, but are not yet ready to show *healthy*, *fertile*, *peaceful*, non-violent, non-traumatic, menstrual blood.

Young girls on the verge of menstruation are sponges for 'cool' so are extremely susceptible to media influences. In a popular magazine marketed to 12 to 15 year old girls, an applicator tampon ad, which appeared in February 2001, assured its readers that while putting in a tampon can be difficult and messy, with their easy applicator, you won't have to touch yourself or get close to any messy tampons. The message is, don't touch, be careful, be sterile, blood is taboo, you couldn't (and shouldn't) possibly enjoy your natural cycle or touching your body.

The lure of beauty, freshness, being in control, 'safety', 'protection', eternal youth, sexuality and perfection are all part of menstrual product advertising. But who is being protected from what? A more honest, responsible and healthy approach would be to encourage girls and women to enjoy their bodies, their cycle, their flow, as a beautiful and healthy part of their own sexuality. Self-enjoyment and a positive self-image remains beautiful and becomes richer with age.

In literature and theatre menstruation is virtually unheard of (unless part of specific 'educational' plays). When it is mentioned, it's usually of the pre-menstrual syndrome that-explains-her-behaviour (ha! ha!) variety. Books on relationships, sex and parenting adolescents often don't mention menstruation at all and, when they do, focus on the physical aspects. Views in specialist books such as those expressed in *The Wise Wound* by Penelope Shuttle and Peter Redgrove, and *Her Blood Is Gold* by Lara Owen and *The Wild Genie* by Alexandra Pope, however, offer a completely different perspective of menstruation — menstruation and the menstrual cycle as an intrinsic and positive aspect of a woman's sexuality, and a fundamental and positive component of sexuality and relationship.

A FEMINIST CURSE

Largely by their silence, feminist writers have also, perhaps unwittingly, preserved the prevailing negative views of menstruation. While researching her book *Female Cycles* Paula Weideger was asked 'Wouldn't it be better to keep silent about menstruation and menopause rather than risk adding ammunition to the sexist arsenal?' (Weideger 1975). Such a question accepts the view that menstruation is bad and, by its nature, makes women weak and less than men (so let's not mention it and it won't be used against us).

Given that women menstruate regularly (and for half their life), menstruation has not received anything like proportional representation in writings about women's lives, power, abuse and relationships. One reason for this may be not wishing to emphasise menstruation and feed the concept that via the hormonal peaks and dips of the menstrual cycle women are unpredictable and variable in their effectiveness so therefore should not be promoted to highly responsible positions or those requiring fine dexterity such as surgery or piloting aeroplanes. Perhaps we have believed these myths for too long.

Pre Menstrual Syndrome?

A recent study gave questionnaires listing pre-menstrual syndrome symptoms, without mentioning 'pre-menstrual syndrome', and omitting any gender specific symptoms (e.g. breast tenderness), to a random sample of men and women, and asked for the frequency of these symptoms over the period of a month. There was no difference between the men and the women in any of their collective responses. Men as a group compared equally to women as a group in their experiences of reduced or increased energy, irritability and other negative moods, back pain, sleeplessness, headaches and confusion. However, amongst the entire sample there was enormous variation between individuals.

A further study that included gender specific symptoms and mentioned 'pre-menstrual syndrome' in the title of the questionnaire had completely different results. Presumably and understandably men were less able to relate to even the same symptoms under a female-specific heading (Tavris 1992).

AN EDUCATIONAL CURSE

Current human development and sex education offers a vastly improved curriculum to the non-existent or highly moralistic and euphemistic education offered earlier last century. Yet current curriculums, in general, do have serious flaws. The main approach to explaining menstruation is strictly physiological, colloquially known as the 'plumbing' approach. This explanation of the menstrual cycle diminishes menstruation to a non-conception, a waste product, an issue of hygiene. Even where this is presented somewhat sensitively and with humour, to lighten up and open up the issue in an age appropriate way, the underlying approach still offers nothing uplifting to the up-and-coming menstruant.

In contrast there are some educators who teach in a way that offers menstruation and the menstrual cycle as a valuable thing in itself, as an essential part of being a woman, of fertility and creativity, regardless of whether a woman chooses to have children. In my own experience since 1990, running training seminars and talking with women individually and in groups about the methods of natural fertility management, women and health professionals are always deeply interested to learn more about the menstrual cycle, about their cycle, and are amazed how much there is to know.

A MEDICAL CURSE

We should look upon the female state as being, as it were, a deformity — though one which occurs in the ordinary course of nature.

Aristotle

In 77AD Pliny the Elder finished his thirty-seven volumes of *Natural History*. This monumental work was a widely read and often cited reference. In it he describes menstrual blood as a deadly poison, which contaminates and decomposes urine, destroys the fertility of seeds, kills insects, withers crops, kills flowers, rots fruit, and blunts knives. He also says that menstruation coinciding with an eclipse of the moon or sun results in irreparable evil. Sexual intercourse with a menstruating woman at such a time, he wrote, can be fatal to a man.

Hippocrates, regarded as the founder of observation based medicine, believed the womb wandered, journeying up to the breastbone, even as far as the throat, becoming frantic when it wasn't fed regularly by semen (some obviously wildly creative observations). He also interpreted the menstrual flow as a natural way to alleviate the monthly distress (headaches, swelling, nervousness, nervous tension and other symptoms) and nature's way of getting rid of bad humours — as neither men nor pregnant women had the periodic mood changes and symptoms, they had no reason to bleed.

This belief in the benefits of menstruation led him to endorse bloodletting as a cure for health problems in men that were similar to those symptoms that he saw periodically relieved in women. From the time of Hippocrates to the beginning of the twentieth century bloodletting was a principal tool of medical practitioners, used to combat acute illness, chronic disease, traumatic injury and even devastating epidemics. Therapeutic bloodletting, however, is thought to have existed well before Hippocrates popularised it — artifacts from Ancient Egypt dated 2500BC depict venesection, most likely performed for healing purposes.

Although there was plenty of health mythology, relatively little was known about the biology of the menstrual cycle until well into the 20th century. It was not known at which point in the cycle conception occurred, or how menstrual blood was formed. Menstruation was an experience that could not be exposed or openly discussed, and relative to other forms of scientific enquiry and endeavour, has long been tainted by negative views and misunderstandings.

Modern science and medicine has certainly cleared many of these erroneous concepts of the physiology of the menstrual cycle and is discovering more and more of its amazing and intricate design and purpose. But not long after menstruation came to be understood as a healthy state and offering no barriers to normal activities, science and medicine also began to explore ways of eliminating this 'unnecessary nuisance' to women (and society). While the scientific approach has lifted aspects of the cultural curse with one hand, with the other it is stripping menstruation of meaning, elevating physiological and energetic linearity over cyclarity.

Dr Coutinho Elsimar, in her book *Is Menstruation Obsolete?*, expressed a not uncommon view that as women were historically pregnant much more frequently than they are now, regular menstruation is an aberration and not 'natural', therefore the Pill should be used to create a 'natural', non-cyclic situation (Elsimar,1999). Drs Charlotte Ellertson and Sarah Thomas suggest that women should eliminate or reduce the number of times they menstruate, for medical and social reasons, that 'menstrual disorders are the leading cause of gynaecological morbidity in the United States and cost industry 8 per cent of its total wage bill in lost productivity', and that the capacity to chemically suppress periods is one of medicine's best-kept secrets (Ellertson and Thomas, 2000). In the US, a pharmaceutical company, Barr Laboratories is at Stage III of a Food and Drug Administration (FDA) trial (2002) for a new brand of pill, Seasonale, which will be marketed for three months' continuous use followed by a seven-day withdrawal bleed, offering women the 'opportunity' to 'menstruate' four times a year instead of twelve or thirteen.

The 'normality' of the menstrual cycle for a great portion of women's lives is apparently overlooked as incidental in medical research into effects of drugs which studies the 'normal' non-cycling adult. Treatment protocols are calculated for these 'normal' adults failing to take into account that a woman at various stages of her cycle responds quite differently to drug therapy as a result of the cyclical changes in her chemistry. The unstated assumption is that the normal human body is a non-cycling body, one which is not subject to such cyclic aberrations as menstruation, hormonal fluctuations, pregnancy, lactation or menopause. It is considered appropriate to exclude such 'abnormal bodies' from medical research on the grounds that they 'contaminate' the results with 'extraneous' variation (and also because of the possible risk to the unborn child if the women become pregnant).

Medical textbooks also often describe menstruation in negative terms. Drawing on a number of currently used medical textbooks, Dr Emily Martin found that when a fertilised egg *does not* implant these texts describe menstruation negatively. The fall in blood progesterone and oestrogen 'deprives' the 'highly developed endometrial lining of its hormonal support', 'constriction' of blood vessels leads to a 'diminished' supply of oxygen and nutrients, and finally 'disintegration starts, the entire lining begins to slough, and the menstrual flow begins.' Blood vessels in the endometrium 'hemorrhage' and the menstrual flow 'consists of this blood mixed with endometrial debris.' The 'loss' of hormonal stimulation causes 'necrosis' (death of tissue). A medical book otherwise noted for its extremely objective and factual descriptions says 'when fertilisation fails to occur, the endometrium is shed, and a new cycle starts. This is why it used to be taught that 'menstruation is the uterus crying for lack of a baby.' (Martin,1999)

This view of menstruation not only carries with it the connotation of a production system that has failed to produce, but also the idea of production gone awry, making products of no use, not to specification, not saleable, waste, scrap. Medical textbooks describing menstruation are full of words like 'degenerate', 'decline', 'withdrawn', 'spasms', 'lack', 'weakened', 'leak' 'deteriorate', 'discharge', 'repair', 'dying', 'ceasing', 'losing', 'denuding' and 'expelling'. These are not neutral terms as they convey failure and dissolution. (Martin,1999)

The following description of male reproductive physiology offers a marked contrast: 'The mechanisms which guide the *remarkable* cellular transformation from spermatid to mature sperm remain uncertain... Perhaps the most *amazing* characteristic of spermatogenesis is its *sheer magnitude*: the normal human male may manufacture several hundred million sperm a day' (my emphasis). No suggestion of waste here although it's well known to researchers who work with male ejaculate that there is also a large proportion of shed cellular material in its composition (Martin,1999).

The view of menstruation as failed production by such authoritative voices from medicine's hallowed halls contributes to our collective negative view. Lack of production is a horror we harbour from the earliest stages of industrialisation and its precursor, the Protestant work ethic.

A change of language may alter our feeling about menstruation: 'A drop in the formerly high levels of progesterone and oestrogen creates the perfect environment for reducing the excess layers of endometrial tissue. Squeezing of capillary blood vessels causes a lower level of oxygen and nutrients and paves the way for a vigorous production of menstrual fluids. As a part of the renewal of the remaining endometrium, the capillaries begin to reopen, contributing some blood and serous fluid to the volume of endometrial material already beginning to flow.' Yes! (Martin,1999)

2. Blessing

I n some cultures menstruation is seen as a blessing — a powerful time, a time to be honoured. In the mysterious ways of shadows, which are wonderfully robust and **will** be expressed, we have already been telling our daughters positive menstrual stories, over and over again, and in this way preparing them for the time when they will pass through this threshold, never to return.

About taboo and seclusion Clarissa Pinkola Estes says in her book *Women Who Run With the Wolves* 'I always laugh when I hear someone quoting early anthropologists who claimed that menstruating women of various tribes were considered "unclean" and forced to leave the village until they were "over it". All women know that even if there were such a forced ritual exile, every single woman, to a woman, would, when her time came, leave the village hanging her head mournfully, at least till she was out of sight, and then suddenly break into a jig down the path, cackling all the way.' (Estes 1992,pg 293).

Even if cultural mores are too deeply imbedded for a full cackle, a break from daily toil is certainly more of a blessing than a curse. It would be far too simplistic to believe that all menstrual taboos are instigated and maintained only by men. Women may have had many sensible reasons for maintaining menstrual seclusion and taboos for their own benefit. Biblical Rachael, for example, while trying to get away from her father with the family gods hidden in her saddle bags, claimed, 'that time', falsely, so as to escape without being searched. This is not to say that the overall view of menstruation and menarche as bad is in any way 'true' or defensible.

In many cultures, menstrual blood is used for empowering charms and amulets, which can be used for good or ill. The Papago from the American Southwest believe that menstruation gives women power and that a menstruating woman participates in rituals to learn how to control and use these powers. Tibetan Buddhist female deities have fierce aspects as well as compassionate, healing and wise ones.

In Navajo puberty ceremonies, a girl chooses a sponsor, a woman who is not her mother, for the qualities that she admires and would like to have herself. Her sponsor carefully dresses her and adorns her with jewellry, then moulds and massages her — the Navajo believe that a girl's body becomes soft again at the time of menarche, as at birth, and that she can be reformed into a beautiful, strong woman. After the moulding ceremony people line up to be touched and shaped by the girl. Through the ceremonial connection to the spiritual origin of her people, she is believed to have acquired Changing Woman's healing power and uses her hands to bless men and women with aches and pains, and babies and children who want to be 'stretched' so that they will grow well.

Although we're used to considering the status of women in India as unequal and less than men, which is true in many significant ways, there are important and intrinsic aspects of Hinduism and Indian culture which revere the feminine and feminine divine and has no parallel in our western Christian heritage. In Hinduism goddesses are at least as numerous as the gods and collectively express a vast range of the feminine character. From the refined artistic, musical and intellectual Saraswati, to the righteous and courageous warrior Durga, the protective and devoted wife Uma, the beautiful and loyal Sita, the fierce rage and destruction of Kali and the benevolent bestower of abundance Lakshmi, to name a few.

Inclusive of and greater than all these characteristics is the reverence given to the divine mother. In India a woman's status increases considerably when she becomes a mother. The force of the universe itself is called Shakti, the primal female energy, as expressed in a woman's potential to give birth — the gift of life, manifestation itself. India was the first democracy to vote in a woman prime minister, Indira Ghandi, who led her country for many years with great support from the people, despite controversy, and was often spoken of as the mother of India. Great respect is also given to the power of righteous feminine wrath (as expressed by Hindu goddesses). Poolan Devi, the bandit queen who was assassinated in New Delhi in July 2001, rose from untouchable bandit to governmental minister, was popularly revered for her vengeful wrath against her high caste rapists and others who participated in the violent suppression of her people.

Many of our fairy tales also have menstrual and menarcheal themes and symbols: seclusion (sleep), flowers (the flowering of fertility and menstrual blood), thirteen as the number which represents the lunar cycle (twelve represents the solar/male cycle), witches as the crones who have access to nature's mysteries, white-red-black themes (relating to the maiden, the fertile woman and the wise crone), stories of seclusion and transformation of pubescent girls. Sleeping Beauty, Beauty and the Beast, Rapunzel, The Red Shoes, The Twelve Swans (the girl who saves her brothers through her silent, vigilant and transformative knitting of nettles is the thirteenth sibling).

In Greek myth, Persephone is abducted at puberty by Hades and taken to the underworld, and only returned to her mother Demeter after she does some convincing pleading and agrees that Persephone will return periodically to be with him in the underworld, at which time the fertility that she lends the world is suspended.

In modern representations of pre-pubescent and pubescent girls we find many stories with themes of otherworldliness, innocence coupled with psychic powers, poltergeists, witches, playing with and experiencing hidden worlds — *The Exorcist; The Secret Garden; The Sand Fairy; Sabrina — The Teenage Witch; The Lion, The Witch and The Wardrobe*. There is something magic about this time when the profound mysteries of life begin to stir, beneath consciousness, to transform girls into those who can co-create and bring forth life from their own bodies.

3. Lifting the curse

I f we continue to consider menstruation as 'the curse' (still our most common and recognisable slang word for menstruation) and behave as if it is one, we in turn curse our daughters.

Based on their beliefs, and own bad experiences, many women may think the curse is inherent in menstruation. But there are also many women who don't experience menstruation as in any way a curse, who enjoy and even relish menstruation and the entire menstrual cycle. So, menstruation can't inherently be a curse.

I was sixteen and anxiously awaiting the arrival of my first period. All my friends had theirs and I had heard a lot from them and knew what to expect. When it came I felt really proud and womanly. I told my friends and finally felt equal to them and all grown up. My first period was light, just a couple of days. Every month after that I had some pain a couple of days before. I liked the tightness, the build up and then the release of menstruation. Right from when it began I have always enjoyed my menstrual cycle. (Elizabeth)

Even if your personal experience of menstruation, which has been shaped by your mother, family, community, friends, church, health professionals and educators, media, partners, and the ongoing unfolding of your own experience, has been difficult or negative, you do have the power to change the collective perception. You can lift the curse and redefine menstruation. Through your own awareness you will offer yourself and your daughter a better experience in a realistic, systematic and effective way. Consider the possible outcome for girls, for women and society, if there were a radical shift of the definition and perception of menstruation — fortunately this process is already well under way, and much has already changed.

So how do you integrate the shadow of menstruation and menstruating women and become empowered and enriched by menstruation rather than diminished by it? Integrating a shadow means bringing it to the light and refusing to vilify it any longer. The details are in individual experience and discovery, the ongoing sharing of these and continuing openness and exploration. A shadow brought to light brings riches, that which had previously been denied and unexplored, and provides rich soul food and inspiration.

By exploring your own experiences of menarche, menstruation, fertility, and the people who influenced you when and how, you will get to know, respect and make friends with your own cycle and body, and give yourself time to honour your cycle and menstruation.

To help your daughter achieve a healthy menstrual attitude you need to provide accurate and positively presented information, have a positive approach and make available a range of holistic therapeutic options for menstrual distress. This will help her become more self aware and empowered with good self-esteem and self-acceptance. She will have healthy cycles without menstrual distress and will learn how to ride her menstrual cycle by knowing the best way to manage her energy and creativity at the various stages of the cycle (for maximum health, creativity and balance). By doing this you will bless your daughter.

Part 3

Rite of Passage

With menarche, you meet your wisdom, with monthly bleeding, you practise your wisdom, and at menopause, you become your wisdom.

North American Indian saying

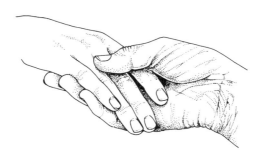

1. Your own experience

How can you be a worthy guide for your daughter as she prepares for and begins her menstrual journey? There are very few Western women who don't think their experience of menarche could have been better, often way, way better. But by reviewing your own experience you can understand the potential of this life threshold and use this knowledge to guide your daughter.

Although the journey itself is theirs, this is a journey for you too — as she begins her menstrual journey you are still most likely travelling yours. There is no one way to 'get it right', no set formula. Menstruation has a long collective legacy as a curse — you won't undo all this in an instant. But through your own processes, insights and willingness to share, you can offer a positive and healthy menarche experience and menstrual journey to your daughter.

First you need to explore how you were prepared for your own menarche, your subsequent early experiences of menstruation and your ongoing experience of menstruation and the menstrual cycle. In doing this you can look at your attitudes around menstruation which you inherited from your family and society. Wherever you find your attitudes and experience don't reflect those you wish for your daughter, you can adjust your attitude and decide what you want for her. Your contemplation, exploration and preparation may be, at each step of the way, joyful and painful alike. You may uncover messy emotions and a shadowy personal and collective history. If you lack confidence in your ability to offer your daughter a clear, positive role model you may hang back or withdraw. But as you take this journey you have the opportunity to see more clearly and by that clarity you become conscious and empowered. This is the blessing you offer your daughter.

By now you already have a wealth of experience of menstruation, fertility and the menstrual cycle, as well as sexuality and relationships. This complex soup of your own experience can be nourishing food for your daughter, and although these experiences may not all be positive, you can offer them to your daughter in a wholesome and enriching way.

No matter how shitty or unexceptional you think your experience, that's where you need to start. Be with it as it is, see what comes up and you'll be surprised. Wherever you are in this process, the robust energy of the grist is what you're able to honestly offer your daughter.

If you've reached menopause, you can still explore your experience. The energy of exploration, the adventure of journeying, gives the creative-life energy underlying the process even as you guide your daughter with more practical matters like buying menstrual products.

STARTING ON YOUR MENSTRUAL JOURNEY

To begin your exploration, find a special notebook and some pens you like using, and make time to answer the following questions. Men too can benefit from this exercise (see second set of questions). Your experiences may be funny, tragic, painful, sweet, embarrassing, confused, shameful, excited, joyful, honoured, awed, blessed, happy, nothing, a combination, or none of these.

You don't need to answer all the questions, just use them as triggers and see what comes up. Be creative. Let your memories, thoughts and feelings flow onto the paper and add to your responses over time as you remember things.

If you're not a notebook writing person, read through the questions and let them trigger your memories. Talk to interested friends and relatives. Ask women about their experiences — most women's stories are untold, and they're *all* worth listening to. Give yourself time and let yourself be surprised.

FOR MOTHERS:

- How did you feel when you first learned about menstruation?
- What was your experience at menarche?
- Where were you when you got your first period?
- How did it feel physically? How did it feel emotionally?
- How did you know that this was the beginning of menstruation?
- What menstrual products did you use and who gave them to you?
- Was there anything surprising about this first time?
- Whom did you tell?
- How did the members of your family react?
- Did your relationship with any of your family change? How?
- What was your mother's experience? Your aunts'? Your grandmothers'?
- Who taught you most about menstruation?
- Who taught you about pads and tampons?
- What was your school's approach to menstruation and the needs of menstruating girls?
- What were you taught in school about menstruation?
- What was your experience of discussing menstruation amongst your school friends?
- What do you wish you knew then but didn't?
- What was/is your parents' attitude to menstruation, spoken and unspoken?
- What is your/your parents' spiritual or religious view of menstruation?
- What is your partner's view of menstruation?

- What are the personal messages you tell yourself about menstruation?
- How have you shared your menstrual needs, concerns and experiences with the boys and men in your life?
- What do you remember from your last period and premenstrum (dreams, emotions, physical symptoms, events)?
- What date did your last period start?
- At what day in your cycle are you now?

FOR FATHERS:

Yes! Your experiences are important too, even and especially if you think you haven't had any and haven't got anything to say.

- As a boy what was your first awareness of menstruation?
- In what ways were menstruation and related issues discussed in your childhood home?
- What information did you gain through which members of your family? Was this helpful?
- What did you learn from your peers? Was this helpful? Was it accurate?
- What information did you gain through your school curriculum? Was this helpful?
- What did you learn from your early girlfriends? Was this helpful?
- How did menstruation and the menstrual cycle impact on your early relationships?
- What is your current experience of menstruation and the menstrual cycle in your relationships with your wife/girlfriend/daughter(s)/ friends/work colleagues?
- What are your feelings and thoughts about your daughter reaching menarche and beginning her fertile years?
- What communication have you had with your daughter about menstruation? What would you like to say or do

when your daughter's first period arrives? What understanding would you like to pass on to your sons about menstruation and the menstrual cycle?

- What is your overall attitude towards menstruation? Has it changed over the years? What caused the change?
- What would you like to know about menstruation? What do you wish you knew about menstruation many years ago?
- What would you like adolescent girls to be taught about boys' experiences during puberty?
- What would you like women to be more informed about and aware of regarding male sexuality?

CHARTING YOUR CYCLE

Getting to know your cycle is an important part of self awareness — charting cycles for several months or more is an ideal way to do this. Charting your cycle will empower you by increasing your self awareness and knowledge. Many women first start charting for contraceptive purposes but before long the rhythms of the cycle itself become interesting and understanding them for contraceptive purposes becomes a byproduct. If you haven't already had experience of charting your cycle you may like to use the charts in Appendix 1 to record your cycle indicators.

Your chart is a sensitive health meter — changes in your personal menstrual cycle can be an early warning of ill health and means of diagnosis. By looking after yourself and caring for yourself menstrually, you're looking after your general health. Charting will also help you get to know when you're fertile so you can choose to avoid or achieve conception (it's important if you're going to use these methods for contraception that you read widely on the subject or get help from a natural fertility management practitioner).

By knowing your own cycle, from the inside out, you're in a good position to guide your daughter with knowledge and wisdom before and after menarche and on into her fertile years. Girls who learn to chart their own cycle, no matter how simply, from menarche or soon after, can *begin* their menstrual journey with awareness of their cyclic physical and emotional changes, and this awareness can unfold and inform them throughout their fertile years.

> Since I was a teenager I had agonisingly painful periods. In my late twenties I started receiving professional help from natural health practitioners and making lifestyle changes. I also began to chart my cycle. The charting, I was surprised to find, was an amazing journey of getting to know this really intrinsic part of my physical, emotional and spiritual self that had been so painful for me. I found it really empowering. It was actually the best thing I ever did for myself.
> (Jenny)

DANCE WITH YOUR CYCLE

To be good role models we all need to care for ourselves compassionately and wisely, particularly if we have menstrual distress. You'll know more of yourself through your own unfolding ever-changing menstrual cycle. So make friends with menstruation. Dance with your menstrual cycles, becoming aware of your rhythms, cycles and needs as an intrinsic part of your spiritual journey and soul life.

Find time to garden (assuming you love gardening). Walk in a beautiful park or bush reserve. Write. Paint. Sew. Sleep and dream. Meditate. Make time to ask yourself 'What do I feel like doing now?', and do just that. You may only have an hour, but an hour of exactly what you feel like is magic, a balm to the soul, utterly refreshing and relaxing. More than an hour can be very nice too. You may find an hour hard won this month, turns magically into two hours next month. Whatever you can manage will be just right.

Make sure you give yourself quiet time and space during menstruation and allow the natural indrawing spirit of this time to guide you. Slowing down is important even if you don't have symptoms screaming for attention and driving you crazy! But if only for this reason you begin to give yourself time, not only will your daughter benefit by your example, but you will benefit as well. And having tasted the benefits you'll discover that by giving yourself a time of rest your creativity and inspiration, sense of balance and well-being, and perhaps also productivity, will actually increase.

2. *Puberty unfolds*

I was not prepared at all when I started menstruating at nine years old and all during my adolescence I had very heavy periods, the blood just poured out of me. Even my first period began with a rush. Luckily I lived over the road from the school and could run home. I was determined when I had a daughter that she would not have the same experience as me.

I started preparing my daughter when she was about seven. She's a kid who loves knowing what's going on and having loads of factual information. So I gradually gave her more and more information and filled in details as she asked questions. I also told her stories from the aboriginal myths and other traditions. Later she got into sending off to magazines for their free samples of pads and tampons. When they arrived we would unwrap them together and look at how to use them. By the time her period did arrive (at twelve years old) she was so familiar with pads and tampons that there was no big deal about using them.

About a year before my daughter's period started I noticed her going through moody-anxious patches that seemed to come at regular intervals, about every seven to eight weeks. Sometimes she had a twinge of pain and would wear a pad just in case. When her period came she had a light flow. We celebrated, gently. I made up some charts for her to mark the days her period starts and other things she notices. Sometimes she fills it in and sometimes she doesn't.

> We have talked about how as psychic beings women's emotions
> build up and that the American Indians believe that at
> menstruation this build-up is released. We have talked about how
> menstruation can be a blessing or a curse, you can love it or hate it,
> and that, quite naturally, your attitude will influence or even dictate
> your experience. (Christine)

There are many individual and family differences in the way girls develop at puberty with some developing much earlier or later than others. As you watch your daughter grow into a woman, the following chart will give you an idea of the milestones — at the same time it's important not to worry if your daughter is developing at a different rate.

Physical changes at puberty

Age 8: Sex hormones, especially oestrogen, begin to surge in a girl's body well before the outer signs of puberty become apparent.

Age 9 to 10: The pelvic bones begin to grow proportionally bigger. Beginning of natural fat deposits on the hips and thighs, and the body shape begins to change, including waist definition. In fact, fat tissue increases about 125% during the two years before menarche to an average of 26 to 28% of a girls body weight. Generally girls need to reach 47.5 kilograms in weight before menstruation can begin. The nipples begin to bud. Some thickening of hair on lower legs often occurs.

Age 10 to 11: The breasts begin to bud. A small amount of sparse soft hair grows on the skin around the external genitals, in the pubic area. A growth spurt begins. This is the time when girls tend to outstrip boys of the same age in height, for a while.

Age 11 to 14: Breasts increase in size and become conical. The nipple area becomes obvious and darker. Rapid growth of the ovaries, uterus, and

---

vagina occurs. The vulva swell. The vagina becomes moist, and some mucus may appear. The pubic hair becomes thicker, pigmented and curly. Some deepening of the voice occurs.

The first menstruation — menarche — occurs (often not the first ovulation which occurs sometime later). A rough rule of thumb is that menarche will occur two years after the first soft appearance of pubic hair. The skin becomes oilier, especially around the chin, nose and forehead. For about half the female population this leads to pimples.

Age 13 to15: The breasts become rounded and reach their adult size and shape. The nipple area becomes raised. The hips become rounder still. The pubic hair is thick, curly and becomes coarser. This is the age of maximum physical growth.

Age 16 to17: Menstrual periods are regular. Pimples have mostly cleared up, save the odd one.

(Cooke and Trickey,1998, Gillooly,1998, Llewellyn-Jones,1989 and Van De Graff and Fox, 1989)

If your daughter is an early developer you may feel she's still a little girl emotionally and intellectually while developing a woman's body and hormonally inspired responses. You'll need to give special consideration to how you manage this with her. While your daughter may be maturing early, this development is normal and she won't need medical intervention to stop or slow down this process — it won't be long before her peers catch up.

Usually girls who develop earlier are considerably less prepared for menarche. So when you begin to see signs of puberty, prepare your daughter for the ongoing changes she'll experience. She may still be your little girl but she does need to know what's going on. Let her know how special she is. She's a pioneer amongst her peers and may well be a support and source of information for them as their turn comes. You could also speak to her class teacher regarding issues of understanding and sensitivity within the school and amongst her classmates, if your daughter is the first in her class to develop signs of puberty.

Some girls develop much later than the average — if this is your daughter it may be perfectly normal for her. If your daughter hasn't started to menstruate by the time she reaches sixteen or seventeen you'll need to see a naturopath or doctor. This is most commonly due to underweight or hormonal imbalance, or perhaps extreme stress (which causes hormonal imbalance). *Rarely*, this is the time when developmental or chromosomal abnormalities are discovered.

Breasts also often grow at different rates, one then the other. A girl (and her mother) may worry about this, but they *will* even out. Some mothers and daughters also get concerned when they discover a lump under the daughter's nipple — this is usually the first sign of budding breasts.

YOUR DAUGHTER'S FEELINGS

Girls vary wildly in their emotional responses to all the hormonal surges washing through their bodies. Some will switch from hysterical joy to deep gloom in a flash. Some will get moody and snappy and others will go on much as usual with little change in their normal emotional pattern. Some just get exhausted and need to sleep more. Most teenagers, girls and boys, need to sleep more than they did just before puberty, and more than adults. But if your daughter is experiencing exhaustion or wild mood swings, these, like all other hormonal or menstrual distress is treatable, and doesn't have to be 'put up with'.

Girls await menarche in particular with many mixed emotions — hope, anxiety, longing, fear, awe, amazement, horror, excitement. Most of us can also probably remember a time when we were ashamed of menstruating, a time when we hid any signs of menstrual blood for fear of being found out. The impact of the secrecy, shame and ignorance around menstruation and the many physical, mental, and emotional changes throughout the menstrual cycle have been shown through studies to have an impact on self-esteem and ongoing menstrual experiences.

As a mother you may have become comfortable with your body and cycle and forgotten any shame you felt. Having a baby may also have wiped out any sense of physical privacy. Although your daughter is growing up in a very different world, all but the most outgoing of them are likely to be feeling some degree of shame. This bleeding can catch them unawares, like all of us, and can cause anxiety that may diminish their spontaneity for a time.

Menarche marks a transition in the risk of depression and anxiety for a girl. Research has found that a certain amount of the depression and anxiety in girls can be attributed to the unaccustomed and unsettled menstrual cycle and accompanying hormones causing emotional havoc.

During the 12 months following menarche research has also found there is an increased incidence of mother/daughter conflict. In a study of adolescent depression and anxiety predictors it was found that for boys the dominant predictor was rising through school levels and high parental educational achievement; for girls the dominant predictor was menarcheal status and experience (Patton, Hibbert and Cartlin,1996).

Amongst the strongest feelings, according to psychotherapists, are those to do with loss of body control and feelings of humiliation. In the end this is perhaps the most difficult barrier for girls to accepting menstruation; having no control over the new bodily function, and not being so many years on from toilet training, whether they remember it consciously or not, they'd rather not go back there.

Rather than discount the extent of any fears or concerns your daughter has, think of them as normal. Providing information is vital — understanding how to manage menstruation and thereby feel in control (as much as possible), as well as having someone to go to who takes their concerns seriously, will make a great difference.

> When my body started changing Mum tried a couple of times to talk to me about what was happening to me and about menstruation and so on. I didn't want to know and would make excuses and get away. Finally she cornered me. We went camping with my brother and Dad and they went off fishing for the afternoon (as instructed by Mum) and I couldn't escape this time. She talked to me about what to expect, about using pads and tampons when I was ready for them, what to do with them when I had used them and so on. I guess I was really glad after all, my period came soon after and at least I knew what was going on and how to handle it. (Jacinta)

Often girls feel it's unfair that boys don't menstruate. You can talk to them, or remind them, about boys having wet dreams and erections neither of which are in their control, at least for some time, and which can happen at embarrassing moments.

Understanding and practical help, being prepared with menstrual supplies, knowing when to expect the next period and perhaps talking through concerns and what to do in different situations (see Parts 4 and 5 Problem Periods and Learning to Ride the Menstrual Cycle) can be extremely helpful at this time.

What do girls think?

A 1984 study of Australian girls revealed they think menstruation is:

- An inconvenient nuisance — 74%
- A part of being a woman — 13%
- Doesn't worry me — 8%
- Dirty or disgusting — 3%
- My body is functioning normally — 1%

(Derek Llewellyn-Jones, 1986)

The Tampax Report, conducted for Tampax Inc. (manufacturers of tampons) by Research and Forecasts, Inc. in 1981 found that:

- one-third of American women were not prepared for menstruation, and two-fifths of them reported their first reaction to it to be a negative one.
- One-quarter of Americans think women cannot function normally at work while menstruating
- One-half of the population thinks that women should not have sexual intercourse while menstruating
- One-third believe that menstruation affects a woman's thinking abilities
- One-third think women should restrict their physical activity during menstruation
- Nearly one-quarter think menstrual pain is all in a woman's head
- 30% of teenagers learn about menstruation at school, while 91% of Americans think school is where menstruation should be taught, but two-thirds think it shouldn't be discussed at home or in the office. *(Northrup,1994)*

4. *Menarche*

Menarche is a wonderful word evocative of a special time — a girl's first period. A time celebrated in many cultures as a rite of passage into a new stage of life with new rights, responsibilities, knowledge, and possibilities — both physical and spiritual.

We hardly ever use the word menarche now and we have little or no tradition and ceremony at this special time. This absence of ceremony seems strange — menarche is such a momentous occasion affecting half the population and marking the beginning of 35 to 40 years or more of menstrual cycling, with the ongoing physical, hormonal, emotional, intellectual and spiritual changes that accompany it.

Commonplace as menstruation is, the transformation of a child's body to one that can bring forth new life is momentous. A girl is unlikely to be planning to have her first child at menarche, nor will her practising-fertility body be likely to be able to conceive or give birth then. This capacity is nonetheless powerful and transforming in and of itself.

All my friends had started their periods before me so they told me a lot, and everything else I learnt from books. I was at my best friend Molly's house when I got my first period. We celebrated and Molly spoilt me with chocolate. I was very proud; getting my period for the first time made me feel feminine. I think it's amazing the way our bodies work. (Rosella, 14)

You may be thinking that menstruation is basic, that there's not much to say, that it's just something women 'have to put up with' and the less said the better, that your daughter will find out soon enough from her friends or when she starts to bleed. You may not have had a good experience and haven't thought about it for years — that's just how it is. You may assume your daughter is getting the information she needs from school or her friends or from books and or magazines. Or you may have given your daughter the facts about sex and plumbing, pads and tampons. But is this enough? Is this what you really want for your daughter?

As you guide your daughter on her journey towards menarche and the menstrual cycle, it's important to be open, creative and honest. Above all, you need to foster an environment where it's easy to communicate about menstruation. If you're uncomfortable, be honest with yourself about it. If you don't know something, give yourself time to find out. If you think you've made 'mistakes', look creatively at what you can do now.

Being open about menstruation from the beginning will encourage curiosity — your daughter will ask questions as they naturally arise and you can answer them in an age appropriate way as you go along. Nevertheless, some girls are more likely to be aware and want to know than others — don't assume that an answer you gave your daughter when she was three or seven will be remembered now. As your daughter approaches menarche it's important to think through what she needs to know and to address the particular concerns she may have. Some girls sport a convincing air of knowing-it-all, and may think that they do. They don't.

Some girls will come to you with all their questions. With other girls you'll need to go to them. Either way, you need to consciously prepare, being aware that as you've been menstruating so long you can forget how much you know and how familiar and comfortable you've become with the whole process. Always minimise 'shoulds' when you talk to your daughter.

As you can't know the day menarche will arrive, you can't plan ahead too much — your daughter may be away on camp or at school or on a sleep-over. But there are things you can do to make sure her transition is positive.

Have a chat about the body changes that are or will be happening. This sort of chat is likely to be ongoing as new things happen to her body, as she thinks of questions and as she hears the weird and wonderful stories from her friends from school. Be prepared for questions to pop up at odd moments. Above all be patient!

Also talk about what actually happens at menarche. Almost always the first period is very light. Remember though that for some girls, their first blood can come in a rush. If this happened to you, there may be a genetic factor and it's a good idea to tell your daughter. Make sure you let your daughter know that menstruation usually lasts between three and seven days.

Talk together about any relevant sex education or menstrual cycle and menstruation lessons at school. What are her friends at school saying? What is the schoolyard culture regarding menstruation? What are the current names for menstruation? Tell her about the names that were around when you were at school. A euphemism I've heard recently for a girl asking another if a third has had her period yet, 'Is she a woman yet?'

Encourage your daughter to know her own body. Let her know it's OK to check out her genitals in a mirror. After all, boys get to see theirs every time they have a wee and many women go through their entire life without actually seeing their external genitalia!

Go to your local library and take out a range of books on puberty and sexual development written for adolescents. Although they may be variable in the quality of their information and presentation they can be good to look at together, as a focus for discussion. Resist the temptation to give your daughter books and then consider the job done. Now, more than ever, she needs your flesh and blood input, experience, adultness and normality!

Talk about your own periods and menstrual cycles. Share as many stories as you know about the menarche experiences of the women in your family or your women friends. Better still have them share their own story. The more varied experiences your daughter has heard the more likely she'll feel OK and 'normal' about her own.

If you've had a particularly difficult time with your periods you may want to tone it down for your daughter. You can talk about what has helped you (if you haven't sought appropriate help, do so now for your own sake, as well as your daughter's). Many girls have considerable fear about period pain from stories they've heard. Make sure you understand the kinds of therapies available and can reassure your daughter that if she has pain it can be treated and she won't have to 'just put up with it'.

Buy a range of menstrual pads that will be suitable for your daughter when she begins to bleed. You may arrange these in a special box or basket and give it to her to keep for her special time. You may like to add some things to the box, like some new feminine underwear, a nice aromatherapy oil, some pot pourri, a diary, a book, whatever seems to suit the occasion to you. The main thing is the pads. Make sure she feels welcome to open the packets, to try some out, alone or with her friends, and to generally familiarise herself. The giving of the box could be a special time and perhaps a time when you can look at the pads together and talk. Most likely she got to play with pads or tampons at an earlier time in her life. They will be taking on new meaning now.

Find out from your daughter's teacher about school policy regarding children needing to go to the toilets whenever they need to. Of course this can, and often is, abused, but for girls menstruating it's imperative for them to know they are able to go to the toilet when they feel the need. Who do girls go to for pads or tampons if they suddenly get their period at school and don't have any supplies? Do they all know this?

Most girls who know about menstruation will be checking for blood for months before their first period arrives. As your daughter approaches her first menstruation it's a good idea for her to take some pads with her in her school bag, overnight bag or on school camps.

While, for obvious reasons, mothers may have the central parental role in preparing their daughters for menstruation, it's important for fathers to stay connected to their daughters at this time. As their bodies and minds are changing rapidly, good old dad or a close male friend as a father figure can provide solid safe masculine support, reflecting back to them that they are OK as they metamorphose into young women.

Make sure the boys in your household are also clued up about menstruation, if they aren't already. Don't assume boys don't need to know about menstruation. They would prefer to have correct information — this will help their understanding of and relationships with girls and women *all their lives.*

Don't forget you can start educating your daughters about menstruation from an early age through fairy stories. By telling these stories you're preparing your daughter for the momentous threshold she's approaching. Much has been written about the power of language and metaphor in telling stories about life, and life stages. You may like to revisit some of these stories or make up your own, adding metaphor and image. Gateways and doorways, transformation and metamorphosis, images like butterflies and Beauty and the Beast, white-red images, waking up, gaining powers and responsibilities, flowers and fertile fields, and newfound abilities to create are common metaphors for menstruation.

For young children, still connected to babyhood and very interested in their own beginnings, menstruation may be explained as Mummy's womb being 'a nest or home for a baby. Blood is the special nourishing food that lines the womb to form a soft velvety warm bed. A baby may only come once or twice or a few times in a Mummy's life and the womb gets ready every month in case a baby wants to come then. When the baby does come it nestles into the soft velvety womb and starts to grow. When the baby does not come after a few days the soft lining is washed away, so that a fresh new lining can be ready the next month' (for families who are preparing for a new baby the story can be elaborated through the pregnancy and beyond).

When your daughter is still young enough to be playing with dolls, consider making some cloth menstrual pads to fit into a favourite doll's knickers (you may need to make the knickers too). I would suggest avoiding Barbie and similar dolls for this exercise as they are anatomically too impossibly thin to represent a menstruating woman.

As time goes on and children grow, information can be added as they ask questions — by the time puberty approaches you can fill in the gaps and handle the practicalities.

A TIME FOR CELEBRATION

Starting to menstruate is very special. So celebrate! Roll out the red carpet! Welcome the new menstruant! If your daughter is not home when her period arrives you can congratulate her, and then celebrate in some way when she gets home. This can be simple — many girls will feel private about their first period so it's important to be appropriate.

I had been expecting my first period for a while and was happy that it had finally come and during the holidays. Mum bought me a necklace and earrings as a present to celebrate. I asked her to tell my dad because I was really embarrassed but he was cool about it. Most girls think that periods are a hassle, but I don't mind, I like feeling like a woman. (Adelaide)

Girls usually become more blasé as they get used to the whole process of menstruation, others are happy to be right out there from the beginning. Allow your daughter to pace the news-telling. She may happily tell family members, or she may rather you do the telling as she focuses on getting used to her new status. Most girls, these days, enjoy sharing the news with their friends, discussing their experiences and giving each other advice. One girl I know wanted to celebrate by inviting all her family and friends to a party at the local yacht club. So that's what they did!

Ways to celebrate your daughter's menarche

- Bake her favourite cake.
- Cook her favourite meal for dinner.
- Allow her to have a day at home from school with you. If you are due at work take the day off to be with her, if you can. Do some things together that you both enjoy. Browse in a bookshop. Shop. Pick flowers. Play music. Cook. Talk — about her dreams, her visions for her life, her values and ideals, her strengths (and yours.)
- Pick, or buy, her some flowers and arrange them in a vase for her room. (What about red roses? Or gerberas? Or tulips or cyclamen in a pot?)
- Choose something that you have that was your mother's, grandmother's or aunt's to give her as a matrilineal heirloom.
- Buy her a special necklace or earrings, a cut above the little girl jewellry she has had to date, budget permitting.
- Work out together where and how she can mark down Day One of her period so she can keep track of when her periods come and when the next one will be due (as she becomes regular). If she doesn't have a diary or suitable calendar to use, buy or make one.
- If she likes to write, buy her a special journal that she can write her dreams, thoughts and ideas in.
- Alert your female family members of your daughter's impending menarche — they may like to have a small symbolic present ready to give her.
- Plan a gathering of women and girls, or just women, who have a special relationship with your daughter, to celebrate with food, dance, music, swimming, camping, singing, fire, painting. Or plan a similar gathering within a year of your daughter's menarche with a group of mothers and similarly aged daughters, as a group celebration.
- A father/daughter dinner out can be a way of celebrating a girl growing up and this being acknowledged by the special man (currently!) in her life.

- In some cultures the dreams that a girl has around the time of her menarche are thought to be significant to her passage through this threshold and prophetic of her future. If telling-dreams is part of your family culture you may like to talk about this tradition or just share dreams at this time.
- Introduce your daughter to some nice, luxurious, indulgent feminine stuff (if you haven't already) — a long bath with a candle and beautiful aromatherapy oils, a manicure, a pedicure, a foot massage, an aromatherapy massage, a face mask (you know the kind of thing!)
- Give her an honest and heartfelt 'congratulations'.

Keep it simple. Be creative-intuitive-inspired.

Some years ago while I was staying with a friend, her twelve-year-old daughter, Sally, came home from school and casually let us know that her period had started. We congratulated her and would have loved to have made a fuss. But a fuss was clearly not welcome. The next day Sally's mum went off to work, and Sally and I stayed home. We spent much of the day talking about periods, and I answered a lot of questions. Sally said she felt especially comfortable talking to me as I lived a long way away and wasn't a part of her everyday life. I bought her a groovy red light for her bedroom as a present and felt honoured to have been with her at this time. (Kirsten)

4. The gear

Choosing which menstrual products to use is very personal. Some women love tampons and hate pads. Some women love pads and hate tampons. Many use a combination of products for different times of the day and for different activities. Like you, your daughter will experiment with different products over the years and find the ones that best suit her needs. If you've settled in with products that suited you a long way back you'll need to take a fresh look at the 'sanitary product' aisle in the supermarket, as well as other products not found in supermarkets. Take your daughter with you. Whatever your views or preferences let her find her own way, but as always you can offer guidance and information and your own experience.

At boarding school we had to queue on a Monday evening at 'The Cupboard' to purchase our menstrual requirements. Before I was a visitor of 'The Cupboard' I was amazed at how nonchalantly the girls would queue up, get their supplies, and wander off without any embarrassment, often using the packs as basketballs as they went. The first few times I queued-up I felt quite mortified and carried a sports bag so that I could hide the pack away. But it wasn't long before I was tossing packs of pads around like everyone else. The pads back then didn't stick to knickers. They were attached front and back to a thin elastic belt. It seemed impossible to get the tension right and the pad would either ride up in front or up in back and one was forever trying to surreptitiously adjust it. A few friends and I decided we would give tampons a try. Between us we bought ourselves a small box of tampons and each took one and headed off to the boarding house toilet cubicles. We were all very giggly and comments like 'I can't get mine in', 'I don't think I've got a hole', 'what angle do you push it?' and 'mine's stuck and it's only half way in' were flying between the cubicles. It was hilarious. Any way we persevered and eventually succeeded. (Diana)

There are basically two types of menstrual products — internal products, including tampons, sponges, diaphragms, reservoir cups, and external products, including reusable cloth pads and disposable pads. There are many kinds of commercial disposable products which come in different materials, shapes and sizes; pads come with wings or without, ultra-thin and 'overnights'; tampons come with or without applicators. Most products are a sanitary white with *black* pads also now available (colours may make pads look less like a medical dressing, but they also contain more chemical dyes).

Although tampons are the product of choice for many teenagers and young women, care needs to be taken. As well as the risk of toxic shock syndrome, tampons absorb all fluids indiscriminately, thus drying the protective natural secretions of the vaginal mucous membrane. In some women this results in vaginal ulcers which may increase bleeding. Fibres from tampons may also cause irritation although most girls and women who choose tampons do find them comfortable.

While toxic shock is rare, it does still happen to some women after tampon use (toxic shock can occur in other instances as well). If your daughter wants to use tampons it's important to be aware of the symptoms, *just in case*. It's especially important to make sure girls using tampons are aware of the dangers and change their tampons at least every four hours.

Toxic shock occurs through tampon use when tampons (especially the super absorbent variety) are left in for too long, or forgotten. The major ingredients in super-absorbent tampons are polyacrylate rayon and polyester magnesium — when these are so concentrated they can enhance the production of the bacterial toxin that leads to toxic shock. Warning signs of toxic shock include:

- sudden fever (usually 102 degrees or more) and vomiting
- diarrhoea
- fainting or near fainting when standing up
- dizziness
- a rash that looks like sunburn.

If the disease advances beyond the initial stage the signs are:

- peeling skin on palms of hands and soles of feet
- paralysis
- gangrene
- loss of fingers and toes.

If signs of toxic shock appear, the tampon should be removed at once (and no more inserted) and a doctor consulted immediately.

Also of concern to many women is that products in the 'sanitary protection' section of supermarket aisles don't list contents or 'ingredients' (except organic cotton tampons). Despite the intimate contact these products have with sensitive, absorbent and moist body tissue, there is no law enforcing manufacturers to list their contents or materials, yet for any other product used inside the body, all ingredients must be listed. These days there isn't much that resembles a natural fibre in or around commercial pads or tampons. For example, the modern ultra thin pads contain the super absorbent chemical, sodium polyacrylate, a salt based chemical that turns into gel when wet.

Of similar concern is the chlorine-bleaching process which produces dioxin as a byproduct. The Food and Drug Authority in the United States has said, 'no level of dioxin is safe'. Dioxin is formed by the paper industry's use of chlorine to bleach wood pulp from brown to white. The bleached pulp is then made into paper products including menstrual pads. According to manufacturers, chlorine bleaching is being phased out for this reason — it's important to be vigilant about the products you use and encourage your daughter to use (not easy when there's no legal obligation by manufacturers to reveal how their products are made or what's in them).

Some women and girls, not happy with commercial products and the messages they carry, concerned about the environment, their health, the cost, and wanting something more personal and comfortable, are making cloth pads again, with modern designs and colours. Cloth pads are usually made from 100% cotton, hemp or organic cotton. One set of cloth pads can last for years, eliminating the late night dash to the supermarket.

Other women and girls are using a small reservoir cup made of soft rubber inserted like a tampon into the vagina to collect menstrual blood (but doesn't look like a tampon). The cup is emptied regularly, washed, dried and reinserted. For where to buy these menstrual products not found in supermarkets (cloth pads, reservoir cups, sponges, organic cotton tampons) see the Resources Section at the end of the book.

Pads and tampons through time

In Athens the goddess Athena was the centre of a menstrual cult in which her 'laundry was washed', meaning her menstrual towels. Ancient Romans and Greeks rolled wool into tampons. Japanese women in the past made rolled paper tampons that were held in place with a cloth sling called a kama. Indonesian women made tampons out of vegetable fibre and North American Indian women lined soft doeskin with absorbent moss. Egyptians pounded papyrus into absorbent fibre to wear next to their body.

!Kung women of the Kalahari desert let menstrual blood gently roll down their thighs and make no effort to conceal menstruation. Men are free to observe women celebrating in their menstrual huts and menstruation is not taboo. Yanomamo women of the Amazon squat on

---

their haunches and allow menstrual blood to drip onto the ground. The women of the Rungus of Borneo also let their blood flow freely during menstruation — rather than using a menstrual product to absorb their blood, they spend their bleeding time sitting on specially dried moss or bamboo slats. When they wish to move around or change positions, they rinse themselves and the moss or slats with water.

Most women of European ancestry, around the world, used cloth or rags to absorb menstrual blood, until disposable products became available early in the twentieth century. They wore numerous layers of petticoats to disguise the bulk of these cloths and to protect against possible leakage. A woman from the Greek Islands told me of her girlhood when, before her period came her mother and aunts sewed and embroidered a set of cloth pads for her to use and care for — this would have been in about 1970. A woman, who grew up in Germany, remembered the hand-knitted cotton pads drying on the clothes line. Scandinavian women traditionally used crocheted pads.

There are many untold stories of ingenious, weird and wonderful inventions of pads and tampons to stem the flow of blood. I imagine creative pioneer women sewing beautiful pads for themselves and their daughters in remote and outback places.

Part 4

Problem Periods

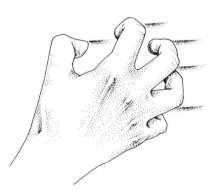

1. *A stress sensitive health meter*

The menstrual cycle is a fluctuating, stress-sensitive, health-meter; a finely balanced, hormonal-endocrine-whole body, cyclic, ever-changing process. The potential for disruption is high and most, if not all, women experience menstrual problems, distress or disruption *sometimes* — many do *every* cycle. It is estimated that up to 75% of women experience some physical and psychological pre-menstrual changes of a mild or intermittent nature which occur 7 to 10 days before they start bleeding and remit once bleeding starts (Angier 1999).

I have always had very painful periods, although some therapies I'm now trying are starting to make a difference. When I was a teenager I was sent to school when I had my period, but would always end up in the sick bay with the nurse calling my mum to come and get me. She didn't have a car and would have to organise our neighbour to drive her to come and get me. I was nauseous, would often throw up and would be bed-ridden for a couple of days each month, but I still felt like a nuisance. All throughout my teen years and twenties I would have to organise my social life around when my period would be coming, unable to say 'yes' to things that would be occurring at the time when I would be a pale shadow, unable to eat, and confined to bed. When it came time to have my babies I found labour a relative breeze as when the pains came they were so familiar I already knew how to ride them through — nothing new there for me! (Jenni)

A healthy attitude towards, and appreciation for, menstruation underpins all approaches to menstrual health. Yet if you experience devastating depression, writhing pain, uncontrollable flooding, irritability, erratic energy levels or other severe menstrual, or menstrual cycle, problems it may seem impossible to have a positive view of menstruation or the menstrual cycle, let alone honestly pass on anything positive to your daughter. But reading the ideas in this book will give you other experiences to consider, ways to process your own experiences and perhaps some new ideas about where you can go and what you can do for yourself. Give yourself time. Rest. Get the support that you need.

THE EFFECT OF THE MIND

Research has found that our health is a fundamental result of the relationship between our mind and body. 'Psychoneuroimmunology' (PNI) is a field of research, founded by Dr Robert Ader, University of Rochester School of Medicine, that describes the intimate relationship between the activity of our brain and the activity of our immune system. PNI research demonstrates the close links between the endocrine system, the central nervous system and the immune system via the messenger molecules, the neuropeptides — a psychosomatic network joins our minds and bodies to create an information system that has a biochemical basis. Bodymind medicine has discovered that the body is a pharmacy stocked and run by the body's own intelligence — the compounds in the interior pharmacy are created as much by our emotions, viewpoints, attitudes, behaviours, and social relationships as by our physiological responses (Lonsdorf, Butler and Brown 1995).

Christiane Northrup in her book *Women's Bodies Women's Wisdom* says that thoughts are biochemical events, that the body and mind are a unity, and that there is no disease that isn't mental and emotional as well as physical, matter being the densest form of spirit and spirit the lightest form of matter. Not only do our physical organs contain receptor sites for the neurochemicals of thought and emotion (the neuropeptides) but our organs and immune systems can themselves manufacture these same chemicals. Our entire body feels and expresses emotion; all parts of us think and feel. Ovaries, and probably the uterus, which have receptor sites that receive messages from the brain and the immune system, make oestrogen and progesterone. These hormones are also neurotransmitters that affect emotions and thoughts (Northrup 1994).

We can no longer think of the mind as being confined to the brain or to the intellect — it exists in every cell of our bodies. So our history of shame and curse can also be experienced as a physical curse. Although we can't say whether an individual woman's pain came before her heritage (however unconscious) of shame and curse, we can say that, on a collective level, the heritage of shame and curse does have a physical effect, to a greater or lesser extent, on all or most women. Every thought has a biochemical equivalent.

To heal our bodies we need to re-enter and re-experience them, and give the body credit for its innate wisdom. Healing, individually and collectively, is certainly possible, through good natural therapies and healthy lifestyle, and through examining and creating positive attitudes toward menstruation, menstruating women, and our menstrual selves.

2. Common menstrual problems

I f your daughter is experiencing cycle or hormonal balance problems they may fit classically into one of the following categories — other problems may not, or may baffle usual treatment protocols. It's important to persevere in getting a correct diagnosis for persistent problems, as well as treatment from a health practitioner or practitioners you and your daughter can relate to and who *helps*.

PREMENSTRUAL SYNDROME (PMS)

Also known as PMT (although PMT generally refers to the emotional and psychological aspects of PMS), PMS encompasses a wide range of symptoms that occur before menstruation, in the luteal phase of the menstrual cycle, after ovulation. The symptoms fall into these general groups:

- PMS-A (for anxiety) characterised by nervous tension, mood swings, irritability, anxiety
- PMS-H (for hypertension) characterised by weight gain, swelling of the extremities, breast tenderness, and abdominal bloating
- PMS-C (for carbohydrate craving) headache, craving for sweets, increasing appetite, heart pounding, fatigue, and dizziness or fainting

- PMS-D (for depression) depression, forgetfulness, crying, confusion and insomnia.

As a parent the main symptom you may notice is *the moods*. Adolescence can be a volatile and exhausting time with surging hormones, mounting school, peer and life pressures as well as expanding expectations. You may also notice PMS 'symptoms' well outside the normal pre-menstrual time frame, such as depression and anxiety — these may simply be worse pre-menstrually. Be careful not to dismiss some of these symptoms as 'just PMS' when there are deeper issues and problems that may need to be dealt with. Adolescents are certainly more prone to depression and anxiety than their juniors as their life is expanding exponentially in all directions — they want to be grown up in one moment and curl up with a teddy the next. While a certain volatility and moodiness is considered normal for many adolescents, if you're concerned, or your alarm bells go off, seek professional help.

Because adolescents can suffer from PMS like the rest of us, good treatment (such as naturopathy, Traditional Chinese Medicine and Ayur-Veda, or other natural therapies), as well as diet and lifestyle adjustments, can make all the difference. You can support your daughter and minimise the negative impact of stresses with the healthy diet, exercise and environment routine, by making time to talk things through, having some fun together and making sure she gets plenty of rest.

I remember one day when I was a teenager my father asked me to go for a walk with him. He wanted to talk to me about my temper and my moods. He didn't understand them and no one else in the family seemed to have moods like mine. I was mortified. I was close to my father as my mother had died when I was five, and I hated to disappoint him, he was such an honourable and gentle man. It was 1935 and no-one understood PMS or had even coined the phrase. I continued to have premenstrual mood and energy swings throughout my adult life, until menopause, and have only recently come to understand what they were. Through the 1950s and 60s such symptoms were all euphemistically referred to as 'housewives syndrome' and most often treated with anti-depressants. (Margaret)

PAINFUL PERIODS (DYSMENORRHOEA)

Dysmenorrhoea can be spasmotic or primary. Spasmotic dysmenorrhoea refers to the sharp, gripping or cramping pains in the lower abdomen that occur just before bleeding, or just as it starts. An imbalance in prostaglandin levels increases muscle spasm and leads to period cramps. This form of dysmenorrhoea is most common in adolescents and young, childless women.

Primary dysmenorrhoea is usually the result of nutrient deficiencies (and not the result of an underlying condition) leading to the familiar imbalances in essential fatty acids and saturated fats, prostaglandins and hormones.

Naturopathy, Traditional Chinese Medicine and Ayur-veda can all be effective treatments. Other natural therapies can also be helpful, according to personal preference.

HEAVY PERIODS (MENORRAHAGIA)

Abnormal bleeding patterns are usually related to prostaglandin and hormonal imbalance. Periods are considered heavy (occurring too often with profuse bleeding) if bleeding is:

- More than seven days
- More often than every 21 days
- Over 80 millilitres or about half a cup per period
- Or, relative to your own normal pattern, if:
    - A period lasts three days *longer* than usual
    - Requires two or more pads or tampons a day *more* than usual

– Arrives five or more days *earlier* than usual.

Naturopathy, Traditional Chinese Medicine and Ayur-veda can all be effective treatments. Other natural therapies can also be helpful, according to personal preference.

IRREGULAR PERIODS

The 'normal' menstrual cycle is about twenty-nine and a half days and, once regularity is established, individual variation a few days either side is quite normal. Irregularity most often occurs because of stress, travel across time zones, ill health, poor diet, dramatic weight changes, fasting or taking drugs (medical or otherwise) and dramatic changes in levels of exercise, usually extending the length of the cycle. If a cycle varies more than a few days each month, or is sometimes very short or very long and is not apparently caused by the above circumstances, it may well be due to hormonal imbalance. The problem may lie with the corpus luteum, the ovaries, the pituitary, the thyroid, or the hypothalamus.

Naturopathy, Traditional Chinese Medicine and Ayur-veda can be effective in improving the natural functioning of the glands and overall hormonal balance as well as the diet, supplements and exercise routine. Other natural therapies can also be helpful, according to personal preference.

ABSENCE OF PERIOD (AMENORRHOEA)

Amenorrhoea is considered primary if a young woman reaches seventeen and has never had a period, or two years past when the other signs of puberty manifested (breasts and pubic hair). Secondary amenorrhoea refers to menstruation which has stopped for more than six months when it was previously fairly regular. Amenorrhoea in adolescents may be a result of:

- excessive exercise
- low body fat
- dramatic weight loss or weight gain
- fasting
- anorexia
- malnutrition
- anaemia
- too much raw food
- stress
- drugs (such as tranquilisers or narcotics)
- pregnancy
- illness
- severe infection
- pelvic inflammatory disease (PID)/genito-urinary infections (GUIs) or sexually transmitted diseases (STDs)
- endocrine dysfunction (in pituitary, adrenal and hypothalamus)
- under active thyroid (hypothyroidism)
- polycystic ovarian disease
- some autoimmune disease

For diagnosis see your doctor and for treatment naturopathy, Traditional Chinese Medicine and Ayur-veda can all be very effective. Other natural therapies can also be helpful, according to personal preference.

OVULATION PAIN (MITTLESCHMERTZ)

Ovulation pain can be sharp twangy pains felt over a short time at ovulation. Usually the pain is felt on alternating sides as the ovaries generally take turns to release an egg. *These pains when mild are quite normal*; but if the pain is severe, it's time to consult a health practitioner as this could indicate the possibility of cysts, endometriosis or Pelvic Inflammatory Disease (although uncommon in teenagers). For diagnosis see your doctor and for treatment naturopathy, Traditional Chinese Medicine and Ayur-veda can all be effective. Other natural therapies can also be helpful, according to personal preference.

POLYCYSTIC OVARIAN DISEASE

Caused by a hormonal imbalance, polycystic ovarian disease (PCOD) can result in irregular menstruation, hair loss, facial hair growth, acne, weight gain, infertility, and cysts on the ovaries. Up to 20% of women have been found, with the use of ultrasound, to have multiple ovarian cysts, but it's only those women who also have additional hormonal irregularities who have polycystic ovarian disease (Trickey 1998).

While the age of menarche may be the same as other girls, those who go on to develop PCOD generally have:

- irregular cycles continuing for several years after menarche
- increased 'masculine' hair growth (hirsutism) before and at menarche
- excess body weight evident before and at menarche.

Comprehensive naturopathic treatment can be effective in treating PCOD.

ENDOMETRIOSIS

Women and girls with endometriosis often experience painful periods and ovulation, painful intercourse, infertility, heavy and irregular bleeding, pain on urination and defecation, fatigue and body aches. These symptoms are a result of endometrial tissue (from the endometrium lining of the uterus shed during menstruation) found in other areas of the body.

Generally endometriosis takes some time to develop and is rarely found in girls during their early menstrual years. Older teenagers with these problems *may* have endometriosis. Seeking a proper diagnosis and appropriate treatment is important — some doctors still consider endometriosis a disease which mainly affects childless women in their 30s so endometriosis may be under-diagnosed in adolescent girls.

An accurate diagnosis of endometriosis can only be made by looking inside the pelvic cavity via laparoscopy (binoculars that look through a 'keyhole' cut in the abdomen) under general anaesthetic. If endometriosis is found the surgeon removes the tissue by burning (with a laser) or cutting it away.

Often painful periods respond well to treatment with naturopathy, Traditional Chinese Medicine and Ayur-veda. Other natural therapies can also be helpful, according to personal preference. With effective treatment many women decide against the invasiveness of laparoscopy.

Are women really iron deficient?

Excessive menstrual bleeding can lead to iron deficiency. Ironically, low iron status can itself be a cause of excessive bleeding and clotting (although it can also inhibit the menstrual flow). It has been estimated that approximately one billion of the world's population have iron deficient anaemia, and that even in more economically advanced societies, 20% of women who menstruate regularly are anaemic. (Donohoe, 1993)

These figures, however, are skewed by the fallacious assumption that women are deficient because they don't have as much iron as obviously fit and healthy males. From around age 20 to 50 women store very little iron due to menstruation and pregnancy, but after menopause iron stores in women increase to similar levels of men the same age.

Dr Mark Donohoe, a medical practitioner specialising in environmental illnesses, says how important it is to avoid iron excess for a long and healthy life. Apparently our bodies go out of their way to protect against too much iron, as it supports free radical reactions, and tends to oxidise or be oxidised.

The paradox is that iron reserves relative to age is the best predictor of cardiovascular disease and death across populations. Accumulation of iron equates with accumulation of oxidative risk, risk of DNA damage, damage to blood vessels and risk of damage by cutting off supplies of oxygen to our hearts and bodies. Iron supplementation to bring women into line with men poses a real risk — high iron levels may kill women at the same rate that it kills men. Women may well live longer partly because they are oxidising less. Iron is very useful if you are charging around killing woolly mammoths, as you need to get oxygen in quickly and have a bit in reserve, but you won't necessarily live a long time. (Donohoe,1993)

This is not to say that iron supplementation is never necessary — many people *are* iron deficient, and girls or women who bleed heavily, or have an iron-poor diet, may be more likely to be anaemic than others. You need to first find out if you, or your daughter, are anaemic. If so, begin professionally supervised iron supplementation, complementing this with trace elements and antioxidants. Always remember that random supplementation can do more harm than good.

3. Treating menstrual problems

I n the last few decades understanding of, and treatment for, menstrual disorders has developed rapidly. The many women who experience some degree of these problems now at least have names for their discomfort. There are also treatments that didn't exist until recently for conditions such as premenstrual tension (PMT), premenstrual syndrome (PMS), dysmennoreah and endometriosis.

Past approaches to menstrual problems included shock treatment for premenstrual 'hysteria' and waving incense at the mouth of the vagina to attract the 'wandering womb' back to its proper place. Even in the 1950s, 60s and 70s menstrual problems, as well as symptoms associated with menopause, were often inelegantly and patronisingly lumped together as 'housewives' syndrome' or 'suburban neurosis', with no treatment options other than valium or hysterectomy.

Despite, and partly because of, the considerable and valuable advances in treatment, the view of menstruation and the menstrual cycle is largely that of a sickness, a disease or a curse, something you 'just have to put up with'. My medical source (who prefers to remain anonymous) expresses the view that the overall medical approach to menstruation is still one of control, with no perceived value in restoring menstruation, or the menstrual cycle, to a natural healthy state. She also comments that the Pill is designed so that the withdrawal bleed occurs between Monday and Friday, clearly an illustration of the almost exclusively male influence in the original and ongoing development of the Pill.

We need instead to think in terms of menstrual *wellness*, a view which needs to be actively promoted by a menstrually aware and appreciative medical profession. Although menstrual cycle difficulties are common and distressing, there are fortunately many effective natural treatments available that harmonise the cycle, without eliminating it, and also allow women to experience the benefits and riches of a healthy menstrual cycle (in all but the most extreme cases). Some of these treatments are outlined in this chapter and Part 5 Learning to Ride the Menstrual Cycle describes self-help strategies you can practise at home to help alleviate some menstrual problems and promote menstrual wellness.

The natural therapies, or therapy groups, mentioned in this book are effective in treating most menstrual and hormonal problems. While philosophically they may differ in detail and language, as far as menstruation is concerned, their clear aim is to redress imbalance and return the menstrual cycle, and hormonal balance, to its natural, healthy and dynamic state.

It's important to give treatments, and lifestyle recommendations, time to work. With many conditions, changes may be experienced very soon, but complete cure is likely to take time in the same way that it took time for the imbalance to develop. Remember that natural therapies take longer than a quick-fix pill because they are working to deeply redress imbalance, not just alleviate symptoms.

NATUROPATHY

The naturopathic approach to health care is aimed at stimulating the body's own ability to heal itself. Expressions of health and disease are considered to be reflections of the dynamic interchange between the physical, mental, social, environmental and spiritual landscape of the individual. The founding principles of naturopathic practice are the healing power of nature (*Vis Medicatrix Nature*), identify and treat the cause (*Tolle Causam*), first do no harm (*Primum Non Nocere*), doctor as teacher (*Docere*), treat the whole person, and prevention.

Naturopaths deal with a wide variety of complaints, and are

qualified to prescribe herbal medicines, homoeopathics, vitamins and minerals, flower essences, give nutritional advice, and perform massages and other remedial body therapies. The naturopathic healing environment aims to empower the individual, to motivate and educate them to restore, maintain and optimise wellness.

Generally speaking the naturopathic approach to menstrual cycle problems is to treat the imbalance and therefore restore a healthy cycle. Naturopaths vary widely in their experience and although they're trained to be general practitioners, by their nature, clinical experience and ongoing training, many do specialise. Seek out a naturopath who has experience and post-graduate training in reproductive health, women's health and fertility.

TRADITIONAL CHINESE MEDICINE

Traditional Chinese Medicine views health as a state of harmony or balance and not just ill health as the absence of health. Like all branches of Chinese medicine, traditional gynaecology has a long history, with writings dating from the Shang Dynasty (1500-1000 BC). Chinese medicine has a profound understanding of and ability to treat menstrual and fertility disorders and uses diagnostic tools including consideration of the flow, or blockage, of energy (qi) in the energetic channels of the body (meridians), qualities of blood and menstrual blood, and the subjective experience of the patient.

Treatment can include acupuncture, massage, cupping (drawing out of stagnant energy), moxibustion (application of heat to specific areas) and use of Chinese herbs as well as lifestyle and dietary suggestions.

The menstrual cycle is viewed as an intrinsic female cycle and one that needs to be understood and supported for both a healthy cycle and a woman's overall health and wellbeing. The onset of periods in a girl is seen poetically as the flowering and flow of Kidney energy (not to be confused with our physical kidneys), when this deep female energy within the body transforms into blood and becomes menstrual blood.

AYUR-VEDA

Ayur-veda originated within the ancient Vedic tradition of India. The Veda was 'discovered' by enlightened seers, men and women, who directly perceived the structures of the universe within their own awareness.

The fundamental healing principle of Ayur-veda is to restore balance in mind, body, and emotions simultaneously by reawakening your own resources of biological intelligence. Ayur-veda understands that the mind and body are intimately connected and that consciousness is inseparably merged with both. The behaviour of molecules and immune cells, for example, can't be predicted solely on a physical basis, but is strongly influenced by our mental and emotional states of consciousness.

The Ayur-vedic system identifies seven types of constitution. Each constitutional type predicts the kind of imbalances that a person may be susceptible to and the individual daily and seasonal routines for each type focus on food, rest, exercise, behaviours and lifestyle. Specific therapeutic modalities (including herbs and massage) are used to restore health and eliminate impediments to good health — the 'same' menstrual disorder may require different treatment for women with different constitutional types.

Ayur-veda views menstruation positively, as intrinsic to the health and happiness of women during their fertile years, and good health and long life in general.

SHIATSU

Shiatsu is a bodywork therapy that focuses on organ meridians (as in acupuncture). Meridians are external energetic manifestations of the visceral organs. In a professional shiatsu treatment light clothing is worn as shiatsu is performed as a leaning pressure. In this way energy and hormonal balances are treated from the external body, non-invasively and sensitively.

Performed by a practitioner shiatsu is a good therapy for hormonal and menstrual disorders as well as general wellbeing.

OTHER THERAPIES

There are many other therapies that can be helpful for menstrual issues — a combination of several may be the best option, according to your, or your daughter's, overall health needs and personality. You may find the following therapies useful:

HOMEOPATHY

KINESIOLOGY

HYPNOTHERAPY

PSYCHOTHERAPY

OSTEOPATHY

CHIROPRACTIC

MASSAGE

REFLEXOLOGY

FLOWER ESSENCES

ORTHOBIONOMY

YOGA

AROMATHERAPY

DANCE THERAPY

MUSIC THERAPY

ART THERAPY

BELLY DANCING

PAINKILLERS

Managing menstrual pain in a holistic way, to balance the imbalance, is the ultimate goal. But while you're getting this together there's no point in you or your daughter suffering agonising pain. If your daughter is not sexually active, your doctor might first recommend a non-steroidal anti-inflammatory drug, which inhibits cramp inducing prostaglandins.

Although painkillers have a valuable place in acute and

compassionate care, avoid using them as your only menstrual pain management, especially if you need them regularly. Find a good health practitioner who will tailor an individual and integrated treatment program to help you eliminate the problem. Kaz Cook and Ruth Trickey's book *Women's Trouble* has a detailed discussion of the various painkillers, which ones are effective for what problems and their side-effects and contraindications.

THE PILL

Prescribing the Pill (in some formulation or other) to adolescents is a common Western medical approach to 'treating', acne, irregular periods (actually quite normal in the first few years of menstruating), painful, heavy or prolonged periods, as well as for contraceptive use.

There are currently three general Pill groups available — monophasic, which are second and third generation progesterones and are the most commonly used; biphasic, which are less commonly used; and triphasic, which are weaker contraceptives and are often used nine weeks on and one week off for certain conditions and by choice (creating a withdrawal bleed once in ten weeks). You will find a comprehensive list of brands and types of the Pill in Ruth Trickey's book *Women, Hormones and The Menstrual Cycle*.

The Pill is a unique drug in that it's designed to interfere with a *healthy bodily function* — fertility itself. There are at least 150 bodily changes caused by taking the Pill (Roberts 1995). If you're faced with this therapeutic option for your daughter you need to be aware of the personal and familial contraindications for using the Pill, including diabetes, blood clots, migraine, adolescents who have been menstruating for less than two years, very irregular menstrual cycles or late menarche, high blood pressure, breast, liver or reproductive organ cancer (or suspected) and depression. 'Major' (life threatening) side effects including increased risk of blood clots, increased risk of heart attacks, higher risk of developing breast cancer, possible link with cancer of the endometrium, cervix, ovaries, liver and lungs. Also don't ignore the 'minor' (not life threatening) side effects which include weight gain, migraine, nausea, decreased immune response, allergic reactions, eye disorders, depression, arrest of bone growth in adolescent girls. You will find complete lists of contraindications in Pill packets, or ask your doctor.

Taking the Pill also causes deficiencies in a large number of nutrients which has a cumulative effect over time. *Natural Fertility* by Francesca Naish has a complete list of these deficiencies.

Although the Pill can alleviate heavy and painful periods in many cases, this is at the expense of the menstrual cycle itself — 'periods' experienced while on the Pill are no more than a withdrawal bleed, except in the case of the mini-Pill where ovulation is still present. So the Pill (and all versions of hormonal, synthetic or otherwise, contraception and cycle disrupters) is contributing to the denial of the intrinsic value of the menstrual cycle. Where the Pill is taken from a young age, especially before the menstrual cycle has had time to become regular, greater difficulty may be experienced later when wanting to reestablish the cycle (Roberts 1995). I know of doctors who explain to their patients how to use the pill to avoid bleeding altogether. On the other hand many women have told me that once they come off the Pill they rejoice in the discovery and experience of their *real* cycle.

The choice to take synthetic hormonal drugs like the Pill may be appropriate for acute conditions — this can then be followed up by a holistic therapeutic approach to eliminate toxins and promote hormonal balance in the long term.

When I was 15 I began having excruciating pain with my periods — I would be sent home from school, or not go to school at all. I would spend hours in bed writhing in pain. My father was a doctor and gave me intravenous valium to relieve the pain, and then when I was 16, put me on the Pill. After that I had very light, pain-free periods but I did gain quite a bit of weight. I went off the Pill at 21 and began managing my periods in other ways. (Jane)

4. Finding professional help

Seeking advice from a doctor can be very helpful for emergency care, symptom relief (as compared to cure) and diagnosis. Painful, heavy and irregular periods are the most common adolescent menstrual problems presented to doctors. Doctors seeing adolescent girls for menstrually related problems will generally start with the simplest treatment and move on from there as necessary. He or she will also consider her overall needs, such as whether she is sexually active.

Most commonly, a treatment trial itself is used as a diagnostic technique. If the treatment doesn't work the next step in diagnosis and treatment will be taken — often referral to a gynaecologist and an invasive procedure like laparoscopy, which involves a general anaesthetic, and further treatment if endometriosis is found.

Many doctors will also consider lifestyle factors and recommend changes. Nutritional supplements, like evening primrose oil and calcium and magnesium, are commonly recommended by doctors these days. Unless a doctor has specific post-graduate training in nutritional and environmental medicine it's better to visit a naturopath for supplements and dietary advice, as this is an area in which they have far greater training and expertise.

Pap tests are not generally necessary for young girls but it's recommended they begin two years from starting sexual activity, and then every two years. Women should examine their breasts from twenty-five years of age, or after a first script of the Pill if this comes before.

When to seek professional help

When you or your daughter:

- Are experiencing menstrual, or premenstrual, distress
- Are experiencing menstrual, or premenstrual, distress that you feel unable to redress at home
- Are needing to use painkillers or other allopathic drugs to manage menstrual, or premenstrual, distress
- Are concerned that some symptoms that you are experiencing may be cyclical (even if not)
- Would like to understand more about the menstrual cycle and maintaining menstrual wellness
- Would like to understand more in order to experience the many positive aspects of menstruation and the menstrual cycle
- Would like help in treating pimples or acne or other 'minor' symptoms of hormonal imbalance that are concerning you
- Would like help with psychological and emotional aspects of menstruation, menstrual distress, approaching menarche, body image issues, eating disorders, depression, anxiety or stress

Persevere in finding health practitioners and therapies that help you, or your daughter, and you'll be well rewarded. Through your own role modelling you can show your daughter the value of being well informed about available therapies and medical treatments, which will enable her to make truly informed choices (even if sometimes you have to dig around for information). Many practitioners now specialise in women's health and fertility, and research continues to reveal more and more useful information and effective therapies. Personal experience from previous patients can often give valuable information about a practitioner or form of therapy. Names and contacts of professional associations that can refer you to a practitioner are listed under Contacts and Resources.

What to look for in a good practitioner

- What are the practitioner's qualifications and professional associations?
- What clinical experience does he or she have?
- Do you and your daughter feel comfortable talking with the practitioner?
- Do you and your daughter feel you can ask questions about your and your daughter's health and treatment, as well as about general menstrual cycle information?
- Do you feel confident in the diagnostic care being taken and with the therapies being prescribed?

Part 5

Learning to Ride the Menstrual Cycle

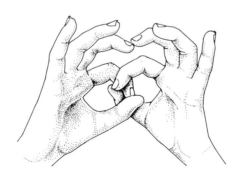

1. Supporting your daughter

aving come through one of her major life thresholds — menarche — your daughter has taken a big step, no matter that it was biologically driven. Menarche is also a threshold for a girl's mother, a major transition in our child, in our mothering, and in our matriline. Your daughter is now ready for greater challenges, responsibilities and new, gradually more adult, experiences. After all, in some cultures she would be getting married and taking on adult responsibilities.

So after menarche how can you continue to support your daughter as she adjusts to her menstrual cycle and the ongoing changes of adolescence? The answer is, of course, very individual and according to your daughter's needs and nature. Keeping the channels of communication that you have set up open and flowing is very important — if your daughter is forthcoming you can ask her how she's going from time to time.

With menstruation comes blossoming intuitive and reflective capacities. The time of menstruation is a less worldly, more soulful time as well as a time for naturally releasing emotions. Support your daughter having a quieter, more secluded, less demanding time at menstruation (if her social calendar allows) and especially if she is intuitively oriented. More than just time out, such a ritual will contribute mightily to her awareness, confidence and power.

Helping your daughter find ways to care for herself when she's menstruating could also include trying different products or offering natural remedies for hormonal and menstrual balance either as self-help or by seeking out professional therapies according to need.

You could encourage her to write down details about her menstrual cycle. For example, on a special chart or calendar she may note down when her period starts and stops. This gives her a sense of how regularly her period is coming, when her next one may be due and how her pattern may be changing over time. She may like to include other things like ovulation twinges, PMS symptoms, mucus, breast changes, food cravings, moods and so on. Even if she is intermittent in her charting, she sees that all these different things change with her menstrual cycle and her awareness is heightened. Similarly, understanding about her cycle will help her understand and learn to manage any cyclic emotional ups and downs she experiences. This might be helpful information for you too!

SEXUALITY

We all know about the ups and downs of relationships and remember the excitement, embarrassment and self-consciousness of adolescence. As interest in boys escalates issues of crushes, relationships, and sexuality start to arise more and more and more. Open, honest and sensitive parents can help a lot. It is my absolute belief that plenty of healthy accurate information about boys, sex and relationships goes a long way to helping adolescents make healthy choices for themselves.

Menstruation, and the menstrual cycle, is an aspect of your daughter's sexuality — it's the first representation of adult female sexuality (not restricted to sex, birth and breastfeeding). A positive experience and attitude to menstruation contributes to a healthy sexuality overall.

Issues of contraception may not arise for years yet, depending on your daughter's age and disposition. If your channels of communication are still open enough for this discussion, and I hope they are, she will benefit enormously from your experience with different forms of contraception. You will be able to offer the kind of information that is never found in brochures. What you don't know you can find out together or your daughter may wish to explore options with her boyfriend. Self-care and self-respect, the value of informed choices and the value of and understanding about a healthy menstrual cycle will all help her make healthy choices about relationships and sexual expression.

BODY IMAGE

Body image issues are rife amongst teenage girls. Although girls and women can take a healthy pleasure in their appearance, based on healthy feelings of vitality, beauty and self-esteem, as a society we seem to have accepted and legitimised feelings of fundamental ugliness, which no plastic surgeon's knife can slice away. Paula Weideger said of her experience of working with women's health that, 'One of the first things I found out in working with women and health is that absolutely every woman, no matter what she looks like, thinks something about her is ugly. In my view, that is closely related to thinking there is something centrally wrong with you — and that thing is menstruation.' (Weideger 1975, in Friday 1981 p.148).

The key life transitional change of puberty has been found to have an impact. Fat tissue increases about 125% in the two years before menarche — association of body dissatisfaction and menstrual distress strongly suggests menstrual cycle changes play a significant role in body image. Attempting to lose weight is significantly associated with increased prevalence of menstrual irregularity and menstrual pain (Cooke and Trickey, 1998 and Carr-Nangle et. al., 1994).

The impact of the media is profound in presenting 'perfect' unattainable images — we're all influenced by these images, to a greater or lesser extent. Studies have shown that women's self-esteem drops after reading fashion magazines and body image issues can create considerable anxiety and lead to eating disorders.

A report on modern day beauty, published in *National Geographic*, found that in 1998 there were 47,000 cosmetic surgery procedures performed on teenage girls, in the United States, including liposuction and breast implants. Many of these girls were receiving their procedure as a graduation present.

You can help counteract media and cultural images by living and promoting a healthy lifestyle. This includes promoting healthy emotional awareness, openness, sharing, warmth and generally having a good time together in your home environment, amongst family, friends and in your community.

It's important you encourage ongoing discussion about the 'ultra-thin' supermodel image and the changing fashions in women's shape over time. In particular, focus on the principle of advertising creating the desire for the unattainable to sell products (for example, the expensive 'firming' cream which uses a photograph of a prepubescent buttock and thigh to advertise it). While you may not be able to eliminate all these images be aware of how they make *you* feel, and encourage your daughter to think about how they make *her* feel. Awareness of the effect does reduce the impact.

It's also useful for girls to be aware that body weight changes with the menstrual cycle and *some* fluid retention naturally occurs (although not necessarily accompanied by discomfort).

PIMPLES AND ACNE

Approximately 50% of girls and 75% of boys will develop pimples, which are caused by increased levels of androgen, thickening the pores of the skin and an increase of sebum (oil). Normal bacteria on the surface of the skin can infect these more vulnerable pores and cause inflammation. Genetics may also influence the likelihood of this happening.

Eating plenty of fresh vegetables, fruit and fibre and very little fat or refined sugar will help, as well as vitamin and mineral supplements and certain herbs prescribed by a naturopath. An anti-bacterial face wash can also help stop pimples from getting infected. A few drops of water-soluble tea-tree oil in warm water will do the trick, or you can try a face pack made of yogurt, honey, lemon, orange juice (add little olive oil for dry skin) and kelp powder (which draws out the impurities) (Trickey 1998).

2. Establishing and maintaining menstrual wellness

Menstrual wellness is an appreciation of the cyclic nature of the menstrual cycle and the changes we experience, physically, mentally, emotionally and *energetically*, as a healthy characteristic of it. Menstrual wellness is also about understanding when the balance of our own cycle is upset and what to do or where to go to restore the balance.

Often imbalance, ill-health or stress presenting in other areas of our lives will be concurrent with menstrual problems. Many health practitioners will routinely inquire about a woman's menstrual cycle when she presents with other problems, as the state of her cycle gives valuable clues to her overall health, and vice versa. In fact, many practitioners will ask a woman to chart her cycle for a time in order to gauge the effectiveness of their treatments and to give indications of which symptoms are cycle related and which are not.

As mothers of teenage girls you will pass on your own approaches to menstrual wellness, and how you care for yourself at this time. This is a wonderful opportunity to learn more about self-care as well as what's available professionally when a cycle is out of balance. You can do a lot at home with nutrition, lifestyle, movement, and self-help treatments to effectively improve hormonal balance and alleviate menstrual distress.

The rule of thumb for when to seek professional help is when you, or your daughter, feel you're putting up with symptoms that you don't feel in control of or able to deal with on your own. Professional help is always given (or should be) in conjunction with things you can do at home, and can be a great step in understanding your own cycle more and how to improve your menstrual experience.

Menstrual health is simply part of a range of at-home diagnostic techniques and therapies you use to deal with the every day ups and downs of your and your family's health. Menstrual problems usually respond well to general good health practices with some additional specific understanding.

You'll easily gain the knowledge and skills to understand the menstrual cycle and help restore and maintain hormonal balance and menstrual wellness, in most circumstances. You may also find it useful, not to mention interesting and fun, to attend some relevant short courses designed for home application such as aromatherapy, herbs, homoeopathy, massage or yoga. You and your daughter may find a course you can enjoy together.

TAKING QUIET TIME

Some quiet time at menstruation is a modern day version of menstrual seclusion. Menstruating women are 'different' and exceedingly open to non-worldly forces — quiet time allows a girl or woman to gently explore the terrain of her psyche, while at the same time allowing her rest from her worldly duties. Quiet time (in whatever form) at menstruation is not just a bit of a break but a timely retreat that nourishes energy levels, mental clarity and balance. It feeds creativity as well as physical and emotional strength for the rest of the cycle, and will certainly help relieve symptoms of menstrual distress.

In our busy work and family life it can certainly be difficult, if not outright impossible, to take days off at menstruation; *however*, within these obvious constraints any amount of time can be extremely valuable, and the *permission* you give yourself and your daughter is invaluable. Interestingly, women in Japan are legally entitled to a day off work when they menstruate.

Adolescent girls may or may not have the inclination for quiet time at menstruation, depending on temperament and perhaps the presence of any menstrual distress. But if you have a family culture of some time off or reduced expectations which value the needs of menstruating women, this is then available for your daughter when she needs it. At the same time it gives her a healthy message about caring for herself at menstruation.

Your daughter may enjoy my suggestions below for quiet time, or may just like to wind back a bit on her busy social or sporting life. You may notice it's a dreamier, more intuitive time for her rather than ambitious and worldly. Through the awareness you bring when you menstruate, you'll be able to help your daughter to tune into her own needs at this time.

How to take quiet time

- Take a daytime nap the day your period comes (blissful!).
- Fill a hot water bottle for the tummy or lower back if you have twinges or soreness there, and just give yourself full permission to take time-out. Ahhhhhhhh!
- Soak in the bath with an aromatherapy oil (nice and warm but not too hot as this can stimulate heavier bleeding).
- Take a long, leisurely walk.
- Write in a menstrual diary — about feelings or events leading up to menstruation and your thoughts and feelings at the time of menstruation. If you're open to writing in a journal, you'll find what comes through at this time will be quite different to any other time.
- Create some unhurried time for creative activity that you enjoy, without a view to any big achievement. This may be cooking, gardening (not heavy), painting, writing, playing music, or craft work.
- Take time to read a nourishing, beautifully written book (or a rubbishy romance if that's what you fancy).

CREATING RITUALS

By creating meaningful and nourishing rituals, however simple, you not only give yourself a precious gift, but in your modelling give your daughter a precious gift as well. Ritual may just be habit, and many rituals happen unconsciously. They become meaningful and powerful by your being conscious and having conscious intention.

Your, or your daughter's, ritual may be as simple as buying your pads/tampons the week before your period is due. You may give yourself a long bath or a long walk. Or find that you like particular food and prepare that for yourself when your period comes, no matter what everyone else is eating. You may fill a hot water bottle and lie down with it on your back or tummy and have an afternoon nap. Yours may be the ritual of forgetting about menstruation the minute it stops until the next time and making a dash to the supermarket for your supplies when you next begin to bleed. Or you may mark the beginning of your period on the calendar to help you stay in touch with your cycle and as a gentle way to let your partner know where you are in your cycle. Perhaps you close the bathroom door and take a long bath with a candle and scented oils to ease the tension in your belly to a soft fullness, drifting and dreaming as you lie soaking. These are all rituals, even if you hadn't previously thought of them as such.

If you were to consciously create some menstrual rituals for yourself, what would they be? Rituals can be very simple and are often best simple. Be creative. What appeals to you? What would you love to do at menstruation? What would your daughter love to do at menstruation? Light a red candle? Buy yourself flowers? Take a slow luxurious bath? Write down your recurring thoughts, actions and practices around menstruation and make a list of what would be most nourishing and meaningful to you. Think about varying your rituals around a theme, allowing for spontaneity and creativity and appropriateness (without too much what-will-they-think kind of appropriateness though!) and encourage your daughter to do the same.

Some favourite menstrual rituals

- Wear something red on your first day of bleeding.
- Buy, or pick, yourself a bunch of flowers, including red ones if you can.
- Put your favourite table cloth on the table.
- Light a red candle.
- Write in a menstrual journal — your thoughts, feelings, experiences, dreams leading up menstruation and now that you are menstruating — it's interesting to see patterns emerge and the insight, ideas and creativity that you have at this time.
- Learn about therapies you can practise at home for menstrual balance and general well-being, such as aromatherapy, yoga, shiatsu self-massage, herbs, the deer exercise, belly dancing. This can become a special part of your menstrual ritual and self-care.
- Take time out. Time for yourself. Unpressured time, time for what you feel like and not from your 'To do' list, nothing deliberately 'purposeful'. Time to dream, and float and be leisurely (even an hour or two 'off' is magic.)
- Meditate, create, sew, knit, do craftwork, write, garden, swim, sing. Change pace. Be inward, intuitive. At work, work at your own pace, use the creative and intuitive powers abundantly available at this time. Don't, at this time, work more than necessary. Don't rush if you can help it. This is the time for labour saving devices and cutting corners.
- Do an emotional review and clean out. Give yourself time to process what has been going on in your life, look at where you're going and what is and is not working for you. Make plans and promise to look after yourself.

NOURISHING THE MENSTRUAL CYCLE

We are so plagued with 'diets', good and bad, that to whisper 'diet' evokes for most of us immediate resistance, as if to military dictatorship, as well as a hidden sense of failure for all the times we intend to eliminate some 'baddie' and didn't quite manage. We need to rethink diet as *nourishment*. Your daughter's approaching menarche, or the early years of her menstrual journey, is an excellent time to brush up on how to nourish a healthy menstrual cycle.

General health guidelines recommend five to seven varieties of vegetable, and up to three pieces of fruit each day, including a varied colour range and varied modes of preparation. This will provide a good range of vitamins, minerals, trace elements, essential fatty acids, anti-oxidants and fibre.

If you make the effort to buy or grow and prepare delicious nourishing food, and this is the mainstay of your family's diet, *then* a little stress-free divergence into fast-food can be a fun thing and probably inevitable for most families with teenagers. If general health is good, this can do no harm — it's probably healthier to be somewhat flexible, than rigidly 'healthy'. But if your daughter is experiencing menstrual problems it may be necessary to stick to closer nutritional guidelines, for a time, as well as get expert help.

Eat fresh

Fresh food freshly prepared offers maximum nutrition. Food grown without chemical fertilisers or pesticides *tastes really good* and offers considerably more nutrition per gram. It also means you don't have to eat chemical residues — maybe just a tiny amount per zucchini, but they add up as the body stores them away for a future health crisis. A number of these chemicals also act as pretend oestrogens and latch onto our oestrogen receptor sites preventing our body-made oestrogens to do their good work. Hormonal imbalances triggered by these imitators affect men as well as women and are rife in our modern world (Colborn,Myers and Dumanoski 1996)

Effort spent finding the best and freshest food locally available will be well-spent *and* economical. Check out organic grocers, organic home-delivery services, food co-ops, as well as permaculture and organic gardening groups. Make friends with vegetable and fruit growers and sharers. Also check out the organic-wholefood variety of convenience food that is becoming more and more available as our collective awareness shifts. You've probably been meaning to revamp the veggie garden for a while — now is a good time.

Oils

There are good oils and bad oils — unsaturated fats and saturated fats. It's wise to reduce consumption of saturated fat by reducing animal fat in the diet — so choose lean meat, and trim fat and chicken skin, where possible. Unsaturated fats, especially the polyunsaturated *essential* fatty acids — the omega-6 and omega-3 group — are very important for our good health. These are best found in linseeds, or linseed (flax seed) oil, oily fish (tuna, salmon, trout, sardines etc.) and oils like safflower, sunflower, walnut, corn, soybean, peanut, canola and olive oils. Monounsaturated fats, the best known being olive oil, also have wonderful benefits. Overall, reduce the consumption of heated oils, add oils just before serving (for example, in salad dressings and uncooked sauces), and add cold-pressed oils of linseed, safflower and canola to the diet.

Carbohydrates

Complex carbohydrates from whole grains and legumes, dried beans and peas, nuts and seeds, soya products and some root vegetables are energy foods and should form a major part of any diet. Grains and legumes include breakfast cereals and muesli, bread, rice, beans, tofu, pasta and potatoes.

Refined carbohydrates are our biggest source of 'empty' foods (minimal nutrition, but lots of kilojoules). Common refined carbo-hydrate products to avoid are white bread, cakes and biscuits and pasta made from white flour. Complex carbohydrates, on the other hand, offer far greater nutrition and can be combined to make up whole proteins (and substitute animal protein).

Some good, easy combinations of carbohydrates, include:

1. Grains with beans: tofu and rice, lentils and rice, tortilla and beans
2. Grains and nuts: peanuts and rice; nut butters and bread; rice and cashews.
3. Beans and seeds: sesame seed paste (tahini) and beans.

(Naish 2001 and Trickey 1998)

Keep yourself informed

I encourage you to read further about food that nourishes and food that doesn't. There are excellent books that go into delicious detail about good nourishment, and specifically good nourishment for menstrual and reproductive health including *Natural Fertility* by Francesca Naish, *Women, Hormones and The Menstrual Cycle* by Ruth Trickey and *The Wild Genie* by Alexandra Pope. These books will delight and inspire you as they explain clearly why eating leafy greens, fish and linseed oil, as well as other important foods, are so essential for menstrual, and overall, wellbeing.

EXERCISE FOR HEALTH

Being fit feels good physically and is good for the mind and the menstrual cycle. Menstrual pain and other menstrual problems are improved with regular exercise. And stress, depression, moodiness and self-esteem are all improved significantly.

Teenage girls are the most likely to dropout of a regular exercise routine of any age group, of either sex. This may be caused in part by body consciousness and anxieties triggered by the changes of puberty and menstruation. The lifestyle habits of parents also have a significant effect on the likelihood of their children maintaining an active lifestyle — active mothers are twice as likely to have active children while active fathers are two and a half times as likely to have active children.

It's important that exercise is a fun and positive experience. You can help to create an exercise friendly environment by promoting incidental, or accidental, exercise (walking to the shops, walking home from the train, walking up and down stairs instead of taking lifts, just mucking around outside with the kids throwing balls and playing games), encouraging and supporting interests in sports, dance, and all sorts of varied *activities*, and making time to enjoy these things yourself. Limit the time spent in front of the television and computer.

As teenage girls are still developing their muscle mass, forms of exercise specifically designed to build muscle (such as weights) are not appropriate, whereas endurance exercise like swimming, jogging, walking, cycling, skating and skills like netball, tennis and dancing are great. Obsession and excessive training can be damaging physically as well as psychologically and commonly interferes with the onset of menstruation and establishment of regular cycles. The key is balance, fun and a positive attitude.

Exercise guidelines while menstruating

- Gentle exercise can help relieve menstrual pain but more rigorous exercise can make it worse. You need to be sensitive to what feels right for you. Regular exercise at other times in the menstrual cycle has been found to relieve menstrual pain and other menstrual problems significantly.
- Rhythmic inward drawing exercise (such as yoga or belly dancing) at menstruation matches the psychological state of this time. You will have heightened awareness of your body which you can use for gaining greater physical skill.
- Avoid sharp, jarring, forms of exercise.
- Cold can worsen menstrual problems, so if you go swimming for example, take precautions to avoid getting cold.

A CLEAN ENVIRONMENT

Unfortunately environmental pollution is endemic and can play havoc with all aspects of our health, including menstrual health. As part of your and your family's delicious nutritious food, fun exercise, and healthy lifestyle program, it's essential to reduce environmental pollution. It's worth staying up to date with environmental issues, new 'clean' products and practices, for your own and your family's wellbeing as well as the health of the planet. Collectively we *can* make a difference.

Use only filtered pure water for cooking and drinking. Avoid buying food in tins, plastic and tetra packs as much as possible and when you do, remove food from packaging as soon as possible. Also avoid food containing preservatives, colourings, flavour enhancers and so on. Fresh and unprocessed is best.

Health and beauty products, including shampoo, toothpaste and makeup) are also full of toxic chemicals. Look for the gorgeous alternatives that use simple, pure ingredients.

To avoid heavy metal contamination use only glass or stainless steel cookware and paper or natural fibre to wrap and store food. Avoid living or working on or near heavy traffic and when receiving dental treatment avoid mercury fillings whenever possible. Dust and fumes from renovation can also cause heavy metal contamination.

To avoid electromagnetic pollution sleep in a room which has no active electrical equipment (water beds, electric blankets, electric clocks, computers etc) — turn any equipment in the bedroom off and pull the plug out before bed. Avoid living or sleeping near transmission towers, power lines, fuse boxes (even on the other side of the wall).

Minimise unnecessary exposure to non-ionising radiation from computers (not LCD screens), mobile phones, microwaves, lasers, televisions, radar and ultraviolet and infrared lights. Consider upgrading your computer as the more modern the computer the less radiation it emits.

Also avoid chemical toxins as much as possible. These are found in pesticides, paint and paint strippers, dry rot and wormwood treatments, glues and solvents, household cleaning agents like oven cleaners, mould treatments, and ammonia based products.

3. Self help therapies

AROMATHERAPY

Aromatherapy uses concentrated essential oils, extracted from plants, that work on physical, emotional and spiritual levels. These essential oils can be applied to the skin, after dilution with carrier oils like almond or apricot kernel. They are absorbed by the skin and travel through the blood stream to be assimilated by the organs to detoxify, balance hormones and tonify the entire system.

Aromatherapy works on the hypothalamus and pituitary gland to affect stress levels, hormone regulation, the body clock and libido. Essential oils can be an effective, as well as pleasurable, treatment especially in conjunction with dietary and lifestyle adjustments, where necessary.

In a professional consultation a qualified aromatherapist (identified as a member of the International Federation of Aromatherapists) will assess individual health needs and will mix a personalised essential and carrier oil blend, administering it in a specific massage treatment. You can then take the personalised blend home to use yourself.

The following mixes, which you can use at home, were created by aromatherapist Melinda Smith. For details about where you can get mixes made up and postal services refer to Contacts and Resources on page 141.

Essential oils in all oil blends are diluted into a carrier oil at a rate of 2.5% which is the equivalent of 50 drops of essential oil to 100 millilitres of carrier oil. You can get bottles for mixing the oils at health food shops or chemists.

Marvellous Menarche Mix

A beautiful mix for a young girl and a lovely mix for celebration, 'shock' and helping a smooth crossing of the menstrual threshold. This is also a good mix for body image issues and happily embracing emerging womanliness.

Into a 25ml bottle of cold-pressed almond oil add:
3 drops of Rose (or Geranium if you can't get Rose)
6 drops of Orange
3 drops of Ylang Ylang

Massage oil clockwise over belly (and hop into a bath if you wish) OR in an oil burner drop a couple of drops each of:
Geranium
Lavender
Ylang Ylang

Heavy Period Mix

This essential oil mix will clear out the liver and works phyto-oestrogenically to balance oestrogen.

Into a 100ml bottle of cold-pressed almond oil add:
15 drops of Cypress
15 drops of Fennel
8 drops of Rosemary
12 drops of Lemon

Massage oil clockwise over belly every day.

This treatment, along with dietary and lifestyle adjustments, should balance out heavy periods within three months.

Painful Period Mix

Into a 100ml bottle of cold-pressed almond oil:

10 drops of Clary Sage
20 drops of Fennel
20 drops of Cypress
10 drops of Lemon

Massage oil clockwise over belly every day.

This treatment, along with dietary and lifestyle adjustments, should balance out painful periods within three months.

Irregular Period Mix

Into a 100 ml bottle of cold-pressed almond oil add:

15 drops of Geranium
15 drops of Fennel
10 drops of Clary Sage
10 drops of Rosemary

Massage oil clockwise over belly every day.

This treatment, along with dietary and lifestyle adjustments, should assist regular periods within one to three months.

Generic PMS and Mood Swing Mix

Into a 50 ml bottle of cold-pressed almond oil add:

5 drops of Geranium
7 drops of Bergamot
3 drops of Ylang Ylang
8 drops of Orange

Massage oil clockwise over belly and chest every day or use a couple of drops each in an oil burner.

This treatment, along with dietary and lifestyle adjustments, should balance out PMS and mood swings.

For pimples

Apply a tiny dab of lavender essential oil neat onto the pimple. Repeat two to three times a day, as necessary. Lavender oil dries out pimples without damaging the skin.

Acne Mix

For puffy or cystic acne:

Use a carrier oil of Jojoba oil, which has anti-bacterial properties and effectively unclogs pores, and Rosehip oil, which stops scarring.

Into a 50 ml bottle of Jojoba and Rosehip oil add:

2 drops of Patchouli
2 drops of Lavender
3 drops of Fennel
3 drops of Geranium

Use three drops in the morning as a moisturiser, after cleansing the skin with a cream cleanser (which will help heal the skin much more quickly). Using the fingertips dab oil onto skin rather than rub.

Dab three drops onto the skin at night.

Bach flowers and other essences

Dr Bach, born in 1886, who trained as an orthodox doctor and then as a homoeopath, reintroduced the ancient system of using flower essences in healing and conscious growth. Bach flowers may be prescribed by a naturopath, homoeopath or other trained health professional, but with some training, they do lend themselves well to home based health care. Bach flowers, and other essences like the Australian Bush Flower Essences, are available in most health food shops and there are many short courses and good books on the subject.

Flower essences can be helpful in treating the psycho-spiritual aspects of puberty and adolescence, and their physical ramifications, as well as being a good supportive therapy used with herbs, dietary and lifestyle changes. You can try these Bach Flower essences:

- Walnut — for the transition of menarche
- Crab apple — for pimples, acne, body image issues, and self disgust or shame about menstruation, supports love and respect for our bodies and menstrual cycle
- Larch — development of confidence
- Mustard — for premenstrual depression
- Impatiens — for premenstrual irritability, impatience and short temper
- Beech — for premenstrual feelings of annoyance with others and nerviness
- Cherry plum — for premenstrual feelings of being out of control
- Holly — for feelings of spiteful anger and hateful thoughts
- Willow — for feelings of self-pity
- Hornbeam —for lethargy, procrastination and not being 'bothered'

SHIATSU

Shiatsu is a bodywork therapy that focuses on organ meridians, the external energetic manifestations of the visceral organs. In a professional shiatsu treatment light clothing is worn and shiatsu is performed as a leaning pressure to treat energy and hormonal imbalances from the external body, non-invasively, and sensitively. Performed by a practitioner shiatsu is a good therapy for hormonal and menstrual disorders as well as general wellbeing. At home you can try the following shiatsu meridian stretches.

MAKKO-HO MERIDIAN STRETCHES

The Makko-ho meridian stretches are an excellent hormone balancing sequence in which all the meridians are stretched and tonified within a whole body context. They provide an easy way of checking your energy balance from one day to another and of working with the hormone changes of the whole menstrual cycle. You will feel refreshed and alert after performing the Makko-Hos. The stretches are also helpful during pregnancy unless there are signs of 'spotting' or a history of miscarriage.

This sequence is easy to memorise and may take as little as twelve minutes to complete. The ease of a stretch varies from day to day and also at different times of the day.

It's important you move into the stretches with an awareness of your breath. This prevents injury and maximises the benefit of the stretch by deeply oxygenating the muscles and internal organs. Generally it's helpful to remember that muscles are elastic and that 'stuck' or tight areas are meaningful parts of our unique personality structures.

Lung and large intestine meridians

Stretches: upper rib cage, arms and back of legs.
Indications: stimulates lymphatic and immune systems, relieves breast tenderness and distention.

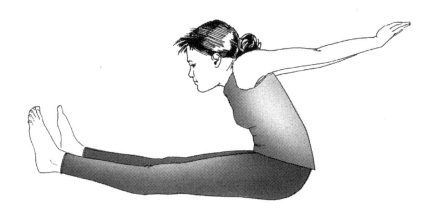

Place your feet at shoulders' width apart, toes pointing forwards. Clasp your thumbs together behind your back. Inhale and look up, opening the top of your chest to the sky. As you exhale lean forwards and raise your arms as far as possible behind and stretching the top area of your chest (Lung Area). Breath freely for 3–4 breaths then bend your elbows and knees and roll your spine upright from the sacrum to the crown of your head, and release your thumbs.

Stomach and spleen meridians

Stretches: the front surface of the body.
Indications: tension in the ovaries, tenderness and distention in the breasts, digestive disturbances.

Kneel on the floor with your heels positioned towards the outsides of your thighs. Place your hands on the floor behind and lean back. When a comfortable stretch is achieved lean back on your elbows or lie back on the floor with arms above your head. Breathe freely for 3–4 breaths. Come up and complete by straightening one leg at a time and shaking it.

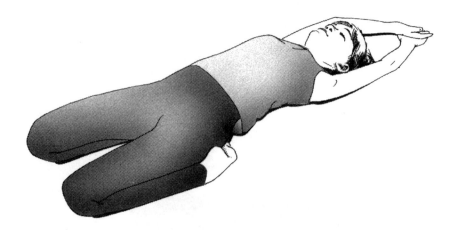

Heart and small intestine meridians

Stretches: insides of thighs and mid-thoracic area
Indications: hypertension, anxiety, mental over-activity, PMS and delayed menstruation.

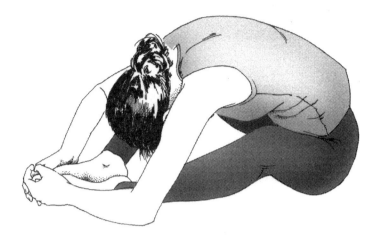

Sit on the floor and place the soles of your feet together. Inhale deeply and as you exhale lean forward. Hold your feet with your hands and allow the weight of your upper body to create the stretch. Breathe freely for 3–4 breaths. To come up, roll your spine straight from the sacrum to the crown of your head.

Kidney and bladder meridians

Stretches: the back surface of the body
Indications: calms the nervous system, relieves PMS and delayed menstruation.

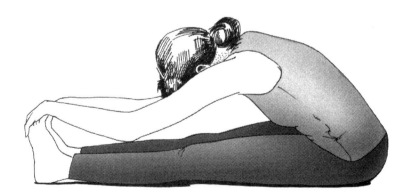

Sit on the floor with your legs together and held straight. Flex your feet so that your achilles tendons and heels are stretched. Press the backs of your knees into the floor. Inhale deeply as you lift your arms above your head then lower your body forward, pressing gently from the sacrum, allowing gravity to create the stretch. Breathe freely for 3–4 breaths then slowly roll up from the base of your spine to the crown of your head.

Heart constrictor and triple heater meridians

Stretches: hips, gluteal muscles, mid-thoracic area
Indications: feelings of chill or heat in the body, tired heaviness (mental or physical), pelvic tension.

Sit cross-legged on the floor, with your feet under your knees. Cross your arms and place your arms on your knees. Inhale deeply and whilst exhaling lean forward so that the weight of your body creates a stretch. Cross your arms further so as to get a full stretch across the mid-thoracic area. Breathe freely for 3–4 breaths. Roll straight from the sacrum to the crown of the head. Swap the crossing of feet and hands and repeat.

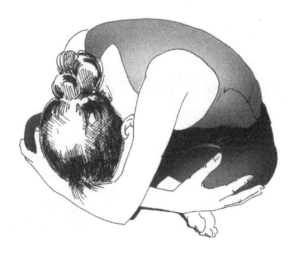

Liver and gall bladder meridians

Stretches: sides of the body and legs, insides of legs

Indications: mood swings, depression, frustration, anger, weepiness, edginess, stiffness in spine and shoulders.

Sit on the floor with your legs stretched apart at a comfortable distance. Maintaining contact with both 'sitting' bones on the floor, inhale deeply and raise one arm over your head. As you exhale lean away from the raised arm to stretch the side of your body. Support your body weight with the other arm in front of you. Breathe freely for 3–4 breaths, allowing the weight of your body to create a natural stretch, inhale deeply and straighten your torso whilst stretching the arm over your head. Release. Shake your legs and repeat to the other side.

Complete the Makko-Ho sequence by lying on the floor, stretching your whole body and gently shaking it.

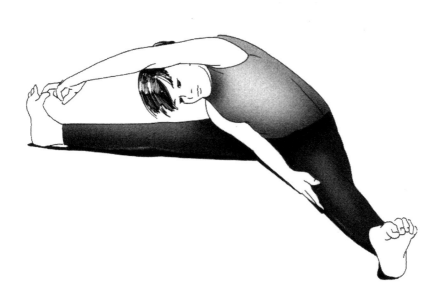

Soft belly meditation

This meditation is utterly simple and great for general relaxation as well as when needing to ease premenstrual tension or moderate menstrual discomfort. It may be more suitable for older girls and women than young girls, depending on temperament, but is still a valuable, simple and portable relaxation tool. It's a good idea to experiment with it yourself before you show your daughter how to do it.

Sit comfortably, whether in a chair or on the floor, with a solid foundation. If in a chair, position your buttocks right at the back of the chair. If on the floor sit on your sitting bones, with your legs crossed comfortably or stretched out in front of you. Allow your spine a gentle two-way stretch — down from the sacrum into the floor and up through the top of your head. Gently rest your back against a firm support. Check for where you're holding tension or are uncomfortable, and adjust to a more open posture. You can also do the soft belly meditation lying down on a supportive surface with a pillow under your knees.

Bring your attention to your natural rhythmic breath; feeling the sensations as you breathe in and breathe out. Feel the rise and fall of your chest. Feel the sensations in your belly as you breathe in and breathe out. As you stay with the sensations of your breath and your belly say to yourself, 'soft belly, soft belly' in rhythm with your breath, for several minutes. Allow your belly to let go more and more, rounding out, softening. Relax.

When you're ready to get up and move about, do so slowly. Stay with the sensations you have generated as you move gently into the everyday.

Yoga

What we do with our bodies for the rest of our cycle will also have an effect on our experience of menstruation. Plenty of good exercise and stretching promotes hormonal balance and prevents or reduces painful periods.

An excellent practice to help general well being, good hormonal balance and resolution of menstrual distress, yoga teaches us to move gently in and out of postures, using the rhythm and flow of the breath, without 'pushing' beyond a comfortable stretch. The focus is on balancing both strength and softness. A yoga routine for adolescents generally needs to be more active and involve flowing movement, rather than static postures.

During menstruation the need for softness is dominant and in yoga practice forward bends are recommended at this time. Forward bends allow the mind, body and emotions to release. Feeling regenerated at menstruation, by allowing a quieter time, and practising forward bends, is profoundly nourishing and spiritually enriching. Different forms of forward bends are suitable for different women and those most suitable for your body can be assessed by a qualified instructor.

The postures given here are very good for women of all ages and are universally beneficial, simple to practise at home with great benefit —receiving personalised instruction from a qualified instructor of course insures maximum benefits.

Budekonasana
(Bound Angle Pose)

This pose is fabulous for releasing menstrual pain (practised throughout the cycle). It allows good blood flow through the pelvis and will help hormonal balance (and the symptoms of PMS), will benefit digestion as it frees the stomach and allows the colon to relax, and assist gentle emotional release.

For best results do this posture alone. There are several ways to practise this pose:

1. To begin, sit on the floor with the soles of your feet together and heels as close to the perineum as possible. To assist in this you can press your toes against a wall, or table leg, and using your hands on the window ledge, or table edge, press up from your sacrum. Breathe freely and remain in this pose only as long as you are comfortable.
2. If you can, practise Budekonasana lying down. Begin as

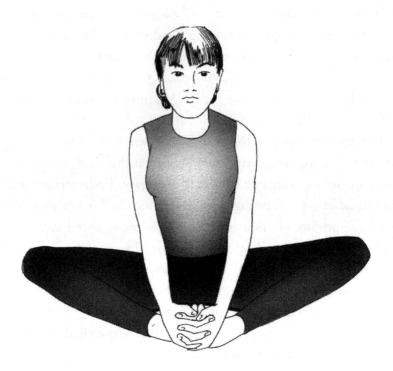

before with your soles together and heels close to the perineum. Lie straight back, with a small rolled neck rest under your neck if necessary, and with the backs of your hands on the floor, about 30 degrees from your body. You can build up your time in this pose as your body becomes more accustomed to it. Five or ten minutes, or longer, two or three times a day, will be of great benefit. To come up out of this pose, place your left hand underneath your left knee and manually lift it over to your right knee as you roll over to the right and come up on your hands and knees before rising.

3. You can also practise this posture with the feet slightly raised, resting on a cushion for instance. This relaxes and softens the pelvic cavity even further and can be very useful for alleviating menstrual pain.

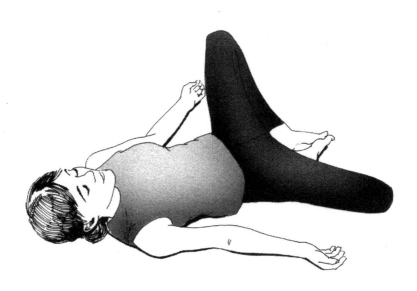

To deepen your relaxation in this pose, throw a blanket over your body once you're in the posture and place a soft scarf over your eyes. Allow your eyes to sink into their sockets, and relax. Breathe freely.

Upavista Konasana
(Seated Angle Pose)

This is also a good pose for promoting hormonal balance and releasing menstrual distress.

1. Sit on your sitting bones with your legs wide apart. Holding the edge of a table, or similar, with your hands pull up from your sacrum.
2. Or, lying on your back with your buttocks right up against a wall place your legs straight up the wall and press heels toward the ceiling. Allow the legs to fall, one to each side, whilst keeping them straight. Place the backs of your hands on the floor about 30 degrees out from your body. Relax and allow gravity to do the work. Breathe freely. When you

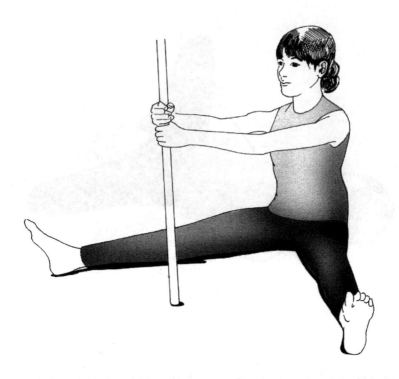

are ready to come up, bring your legs up the wall to meet and then bend knees to press them into your chest, roll to the right to come up. (This variation is called Supta Vista Konasana.)

The Blessing

There was once a king and queen who had been married for many years. At long last a child was born to them and they named her Briar Rose. At her baptism they decided to hold a great celebration and amongst the guests to be invited would be the wise women of the realm who had power to bestow upon the princess special gifts. There were thirteen wise women but the king and queen had only twelve gold plates so they decided not to ask the thirteenth — but she came anyway, uninvited.

At the feast each of the wise women conferred on the baby princess their gifts. The thirteenth wise woman came out of the shadows, causing a ripple to pass through the assembly. 'My gift is the greatest of them all,' she said, her voice cracking like lightening. 'On her thirteenth birthday the child will prick herself with a spindle and die.' Led by the king, there was a great gasp from the assembly.

The king decreed that every spindle in the realm and every object that could draw blood be destroyed. Great fires burned as the king destroyed all possibility that the curse of the thirteenth wise woman's would come true.

Briar Rose enjoyed a happy childhood roaming the palace, studying dancing, singing, languages, algebra and philosophy and was loved by all who knew her. On the day of her thirteenth birthday she was feeling strangely restless and decided to explore a part of the castle that she had never explored before. She followed the steps as far as they would go until she came to an old wooden door. She reached out to push it but before her hand touched the door it opened by itself. 'Come in', said the voice of an old woman who was sitting spinning. The curious girl entered and as soon as she stepped over the threshold she discovered that she was bleeding. She thought it very odd because she hadn't touched anything, and the blood wasn't coming from her hand. She entered the room and the door closed forever behind her.

Then the thirteenth wise woman, for it was she who was spinning the fabric of life, explained to the woman newly emerged from the girl, the mysteries of the body that bleeds but is not wounded. And she lived happily ever after.

Appendix

CHARTING YOUR MENSTRUAL CYCLE — FOR MOTHERS AND DAUGHTERS

Using the *menstrual cycle chart* (page 139) you can fill in the menstrual cycle symptoms and changes that are relevant for you. First make photocopies of the blank chart, or scan it onto your computer, and then fill in the *symptoms and changes column* from the list below, adding others if you wish.

Use colours or symbols to indicate qualities and shading up to a certain level in a box to indicate quantities. Use a tick or other symbol to indicate something is present, but leave the box empty if it is not present to avoid an overly full chart. You can enter the colour/symbol you have chosen for each of the items in the *colour/symbol column*.

Symptoms and changes to chose from:

- Bleeding (menstrual and spotting) — use colours or symbols to indicate quantity, colour, spotting, clots and so on
- Pain— menstrual, mid-cycle, or other
- Cervical mucus as found at the vaginal opening — use colours or symbols to indicate quantity and quality.
- Position of cervix — high or low
- Feeling bloated
- Sore breasts
- Food cravings — use symbols to indicate different cravings
- Headaches

- Oily hair
- Pimples
- Energy — use colours or symbols for different qualities of energy like high, low, ragged, nervous, lethargic, harmonious, flowing and so on.
- Moods — use colours or symbols for different moods like sad, lonely, angry, irritable, anxious, happy, peaceful, inspired, lonely, self-contained, creative, dreamy.
- Dreams — use symbols to indicate healing, disturbing, funny, good or bad dreams.
- Romantic thoughts and feelings about boys you know, movie stars or rock stars.
- Moon phase at day one of your cycle.
- What other symptoms and changes do you think may be relevant to your menstrual cycle?

After even just a couple of months you will find the patterns of your own cycle emerging. This will give you valuable information about how best to look after and pace yourself during your cycle.

The *menstrual calendar* (page 140) is a generic annual calendar you can copy and use to record your periods and ovulation, or approximate ovulation, if known. As you fill in the calendar you will be able to see at a glance the pattern of your menstrual cycle over the year, it's regularity/irregularity, when your next period is due and so on.

Date on first day of cycle (menstruation):

Symptoms and changes	Symbols colours	1	2	3	4	5	6	7	8	9	10	11	12	13	14	15	16	17	18	19	20	21	22	23	24	25	26	27	28	29	30	31	32	33	34	35

The menstrual cycle chart

MONTH \ DAY	1	2	3	4	5	6	7	8	9	10	11	12	13	14	15	16	17	18	19	20	21	22	23	24	25	26	27	28	29	30	31
January																															
February																													▨	▨	
March																														▨	
April																														▨	
May																															
June																															
July																															
August																														▨	
September																															
October																														▨	
November																															
December																															

The menstrual calendar

140

Contacts and resources

MENSTRUAL PRODUCTS

Australia
Rad-Pads
100% cotton cloth pads
PO Box 786
Castlemaine
VIC 3450
Ph: 03 54724922
Fax: 03 54705766
Website: www.radpads.com.au

Moonphase Period Piece
100% cotton cloth pads
PO Box 1018
Bondi Junction
NSW 1355
Ph/fax: 02 9310 0591
Email: aepope@ozemail.com.au

Wise Woman Cloths
Organic cloth pads
PO Box 250
Canterbury
VIC 3126
Ph/fax: 03 9830 5280

Wemoon
Cloth pads
PO Box 249
Byron Bay
NSW 2481
Ph: 02 6684 6300

The Keeper
Rubber reservoir cup
PO Box 305
Bundanoon
NSW 2578
Email: keepercup@hotmail.com
Website: www.keeper.com.au

Sea Sponge Tampons
Chemists and pharmacies
Buy sea sponges that are used
for removing makeup (not
loofahs!), choose a size and
shape that seems suitable and
thread a needle with embroidery
cotton or silk, run the thread up
through the middle of the
sponge-tampon and down again,
remove needle and tie a knot at

the end. Use the thread as the tampon 'string' to help remove it. Wash and dry carefully. Adding tea-tree oil to the last rinse adds freshness.

Organic Cotton Tampons

Available in health food shops and some supermarkets.
You can make your own cloth pads. Get creative and experiment.

New Zealand
Moontime Aotearoa

100% Cotton Cloth Pads
Luna Collective for Women's Wellness
PO Box 836
Nelson
Ph/fax: 03 5458505
Email: lunacollective@ts.co.nz
Website: www.luna.tasman.net

Available in most health food shops around New Zealand

The Keeper

PO Box 47820
Ponsonby
Auckland

Sea Sponge Tampons

Maree Hassick
Waiora Mara
Pokororo, RD 1
Motueka
Ph: 03 5268829

United Kingdom
Ecofemme UK

100% Cotton Cloth Pads
Dominique Pahud
15 Holmesdale Road
Bristol, BS3 4QL
Ph: 0117 904 9726
Email: dompahud@hotmail.com

Feminine Alternatives

Cloth pads, sponges, menstrual cycle information
18 Tor View Avenue
Glastonbury
Somerset BA6 8AF
Ph: 01458 834787

Natracare Feminine Hygiene

Unbleached and chemical free tampons and pads
C/- Bodywise (UK) Ltd
Bristol BS32 4DX
Ph: 0145 461 5500
Email: info@natracare.com

United States
Menstrual Health Foundation
Cloth Pads and other related products
PMB# 181
Sebastopol
California 95472
Ph: 707 522 8662
Fax: 707 823 2137
Website: www.cyclesinc.org

Moonflower Natural Products Catalogue
Cloth Pads
141 Commercial St NE
Salem
OR 97301
Ph: 503 371445
Fax: 503 371 5395
FREECALL 1800 443 9942
Website: www.1CASCADE.com

Gladrags
Cloth Pads
PO Box 12648
Portland
OR 97212
Ph: 503 282 0436
FREECALL 1800 799 GLAD
Email: b@gladrags.com

OTHER RELATED PRODUCTS

Moon Charts
Annual Moon Chart Calendar
PO Box 40
Ainslie
ACT 2602
Ph: 02 6248 7225
Website: www.moonchart.com.au

Moon Diary Products
Annual Moon Cycle Calendar and Moon Diary
Po Box 421
Bellingen
NSW 2454
Ph/fax: 02 6655 2536
Email: sales@moondiary.com.au
Website: www.moondiary.com.au

The Perfect Potion
Offers personal Aromatherapy blends and a mail order service
Ph: 07 3256 8500
Fax: 07 3256 8600
Website: www.perfectpotion.com.au

United Kingdom
The Moon Calendar Company
PO Box 2477
Bradford-on-Avon BA15 2XY
Ph: 0122 586 8850
Website: www.mooncalendar.co.uk

143

Natural Parent

Magazine for holistic family living
4 Wallace Road
London N1 2PG
Ph: 0171 354 4592
Email: wddty@zoo.co.uk

United States
New Moon

The Magazine for Girls and
Their Dreams
Has no advertising and includes
stories of rites of passage,
different cultural experiences, and
menarche.
P.O. Box 3587
Duluth
MN 55803-3587, U.S.A.
Website: www.newmoon.org

WORKSHOPS AND COURSES

Jane Bennett

PO Box 786
Castlemaine
VIC 3450
ph: 03 54724922
fax: 03 54705766
email: jane@fertility.com.au
I offer A Blessing Not A Curse
one-day workshops for mothers
and daughters, and half- day
seminars for health, teaching and
welfare professionals.

Sue Laing

Healthy Living Australia
104c Longwood Road
Heathfield
SA 5153
ph: 08 8339 4412
Sue runs Children and Sexuality
courses for parents which are
aimed at helping parents answer
children's questions and travels
widely to do so. Call to check her
current itinerary or you can offer
to organise a group in your area.
Individual consultations also
available.

Alexandra Pope

PO Box 1018
Bondi Junction
NSW 1355
Ph/fax: 02 9310 0591
Email: aepope@ozemail.com.au
Author of *The Wild Genie*,
Alexandra is a psychotherapist
and offers workshops for women
on menstrual health and female
power.

Amrita Hobbs

PO Box 337
Kyogle
NSW 2474
Ph: 0419 336291
Email: amritahobbs@bigpond.com

Amrita runs workshops in Australia and overseas to support girls and women through key life massages. Current programs include: Girls Growing Up (mother and daughter and father and daughter); Rites of Passage (for teenagers); Reclaiming First Rites (for women).

Shushann Movsessian

ph: 02 9386 5642
email: shushann@ozemail.com.au
Shushann offers puberty workshops for girls from 9–12 as well as parent and mother and daughter programs.

Felicity Oswell

PO Box 206
Manly
NSW 1655
Ph: 02 9983 9440

Felicity runs Mandala Moon workshops in Australia and Japan using art and dance, as well as leading and teaching the Mandala Dance of the Twenty-one Taras and develops Wisdom Moon programs for women focusing on cyclic and menstrual awareness.

Kerry Hampton

PO Box 250
Canterbury
Vic 3126
Ph/fax: 03 9830 5280
Kerry offers fertility awareness tuition, menstrual cycle education and mother and daughter evenings.

The International College of Spiritual Midwifery

Level 1, 210 Lonsdale Street
Melbourne
Vic 3000
Ph/fax: 03 9654 3737
Offers a range of seminars and workshops including adolescent programs.

New Zealand
The Health Alternatives for Women (THAW)

A health information and resource centre, including menstrual cycle information
PO Box 884
Christchurch
Ph: 03 379 6970
Fax: 03 366 3470
Email: thaw@ch.planet.gen.nz

United Kingdom
Cabby Laffy
Cabby offers individual and group sessions and workshops on fertility and/or sexuality, providing practical and emotional support.
Ph: 020 7482 6371
Email: cabbylaffy@yahoo.co.uk

Dominique Kerr
Menarche educator
Ph: 0117 904 9726

Katheryn Trenshaw
Offers workshops and courses on women's mysteries
PO Box 3 TOTNES
Devon TQ95LT
Ph/fax: 01803 863 553
Email: post@ktrenshaw.com
Website: www.ktrenshaw.com

United States
Menstrual Health Foundation
Tamara Slayton
708 Gravenstein Hwy North
PMB #181
Sebastopol
California 95472
Ph: 707 522 8662
Fax: 707 823 2137
Website: www.cyclesinc.org

Tamara offers educational programs on coming of age, menstruation and fertility cycles, menopause, teacher training, curriculum development and program design. Online courses available.

Judith Barr
PO Box 218
North Salem
New York 10560
Ph/fax: 914 669 5822
Email: judbarr@judithbarr.com
Website: www.judithbarr.com
Judith works with individuals and groups worldwide teaching on the feminine and women's mysteries, including workshops on menstruation, menopause and sexuality.

PROFESSIONAL ASSOCIATIONS

Australia
For a qualified professional in your area you can contact:

International Federation of Aromatherapists
PO Box 635
Albert Street
Brisbane 4002
Ph: 07 3012 8160

Australian Association of Reflexology
Ph: 02 43622795

Association of Massage Therapists Australia Inc.
PO Box 627
South Yarra
VIC 3141
FREECALL 1800 353 930
Ph: 03 95103930
Website: www.amta.asn.au

Association of Remedial Masseurs
1/20 Blaxland Road
Ryde
NSW 2112
Ph: 02 98074769

Australian Acupuncture and Chinese Medicine Association Ltd.
PO Box 5142
West End
QLD 4101
FREECALL 1800 025 334
Ph: 07 38465866

Natural Herbalists Association of Australia
PO Box 61
Broadway
NSW 2007

Ph: 02 9560 7077

The Shiatsu Therapists Association of Australia
PO Box 598
Belgrave
VIC 3160
Ph/fax: 03 97526711

Australian Society of Clinical Hypnotherapists
30 Denistone Road
Eastwood
NSW 2122
Ph: 02 9874 2776
Website: www.asch.com.au

Australian Natural Therapists Association
PO Box A964
Sydney
NSW 2000
Ph: 02 92832234
Country and interstate:
1800 817 577

Australian Traditional Medicine Association
PO Box 1027
Meadowbank
NSW 2114
Ph: 02 9809 6800

New Zealand

Shiatsu Practitioners Association Aotearoa
Desiree Bailey
365 Ngatai Road
Otumoetai
Tauranga
Ph: 07 570 0188

New Zealand Association of Therapeutic Massage Practitioners
PO Box 375
Hamilton
Email: nzatmp@ihug.co.nz

New Zealand Charter of Health Practitioners Inc.
PO Box 36588
Northcote
Auckland
Ph: 09 4436255

New Zealand Register of Acupuncturists Inc.
PO Box 9950
Wellington
Ph: 08 00228786
Email: nzra@acupuncture.org.nz

South Pacific Association of Natural Therapists
28 Willow Avenue
Birkenhead
Auckland
Ph/fax: 09 4809 089

United Kingdom

The British Acupuncture Council
Park House
206-208 Latimer Road
London W10 6RE
Ph: 020 8964 0222

Professional Register of Traditional Chinese Medicine
100 Marlborough Road
Dublin 4
Ph: 01 496 7830

International Federation of Aromatherapists
Stamford House
2/4 Chiswick High Road
London W4 1TH
Ph: 020 8742 2605

The Ayurvedic Company of Great Britain
50 Penywern Road
London SW5 9SX
Ph: 020 7370 2255

The British Herbal Medicine Association

Sun House
Church Street
Stroud
Gloucestershire GL5 1JL
Ph: 0145 375 1389

General Council of Naturopathy

Goswell House
2 Goswell Road
Somerset BA16 OJG
Ph: 01458 840072
Website: www.naturopathy.org.uk

Society of Homoeopaths

4a Artizan Road
Northhampton NN1 4HN
Ph: 0160 462 1400

General Council of Osteopathy

Osteopathy House
176 Tower Bridge Road
London SE1 3OU
Ph: 020 7357 6655

The European Shiatsu Network

Highbanks
Lockeridge, Marlborough
Wiltshire SN8 4EQ
Ph: 0167 286 1362

The Dr Bach Foundation

Mount Vernon
Sotwell
Wallingford
Oxon OX10 OP2
Ph: 0149 183 4678

United States

The American Association of Naturopathic Physicians

PO Box 20386
Seattle WA 98112
Ph: 206 298 0125

The American Holistic Medical Association

6728 Old McLean Village Drive
McLean,
VA 22101
Ph: 703 556 9245

American Herbalists Guild

PO Box 746555
Arvada
CO 80006
Ph: 303 423 8800

Northeast Herbal Association

PO Box 146
Marshfield
VT 05658
Ph: 802 456 1402

THERAPISTS

Australia
Natural Fertility Management

The Jocelyn Centre for Natural Fertility Management and Holistic Medicine
46 Grosvenor Street
Woollahra
NSW 2025
Ph: 02 93692047
Email: enquiries@fertility.com.au
Website: www.fertility.com.au
The Jocelyn Centre, founded by Francesca Naish, offers comprehensive naturopathic care for menstrual cycle, hormonal and reproductive problems as well as the Natural Fertility Management methods of fertility awareness for use throughout a woman's fertile life for effective contraception and conscious conception. Also available: Natural Fertility Management Kits. Phone or write for a brochure or order form, or you can download an order form from the website.

Natural Fertility Management Counsellors

For the closest health professional to you who has trained with Francesca Naish and is accredited as a Natural Fertility Management Counsellor:
Ph: 02 93692047

Dorothy Douglas

70 Croydon Road
Croydon
VIC 3136
Ph: 03 97233933
Dorothy offers 'Shiatsu for Yourself' classes where you can learn meridian stretches and self-massage. Dorothy is also available for individual therapy sessions.

Alexandra Pope

Counselling and psychotherapy, specialising in menstrual health and menopause.
PO Box 1018
Bondi Junction
NSW 1355
Ph/fax: 02 9310 0591
Email: aepope@ozemail.com.au

New Zealand
Natural Fertility Management Counsellors
Jo Barnett
39 Trent Street
Christchurch
Ph: 03 381 4924
Email: jo.barnett@paradise.net.nz

United States
Joyce Stahmann
Natural Fertility Management
Counsellor and herbalist
Email: stahmann@yahoo.com
Website: www.herbalwellness.net

SUPPORT GROUPS, ASSOCIATIONS AND INFORMATION SERVICES

Australia
Women's Information Referral Centre
Level 1, Block A
Callam Offices
Woden ACT 2606
Ph: 02 6205 1075
Fax: 02 6205 1077

Women's Information and Referral Service
Department for Women
Level 11, 100 William Street
Woolloomooloo
NSW 2011
Ph: 02 93341047
FREECALL 1800 817 227
Fax: 02 93341023

Women's Information Network
PO Box 40596
Casuarina
NT 0811
Ph: 08 8922 7276
FREECALL 1800 813 631

Women's Information Centre
Cnr Gregory and Bath Streets
Alice Springs
NT 0870
Ph: 08 8951 5880
Fax: 08 8951 5884

Women's Information Link
56 Mary Street
Brisbane
QLD 4000
Postal: PO Box 316,
Brisbane,
QLD 4000

Ph: 07 3224 2211
FREECALL 1800 177 577
Fax: 1800 656 122

Women's Information and Referral Service
230 Mulgrave Street
Cairns
QLD 4870
Ph: 07 4051 9366

Women's Information Service
122 Kintore Avenue
Adelaide
SA 5000
Ph: 08 8207 7677
FREECALL 1800 188 158
Fax: 08 8207 7676

Women's Information and Referral Exchange
1st Floor, 247 Flinders Lane
Melbourne
VIC 3000
Ph: 03 9654 6844
FREECALL 1800 136 570
Fax: 03 9654 6831
Email: wire@vicnet.net.au
Website: www.vicnet.net.au/-wire

Women's Information Service
1st Floor, West Australia Square
141 St George's Terrace
Perth
WA 6000
Ph: 08 9264 1900
FREECALL 1800 199 174
Fax: 08 9264 1925

Endometriosis Association of NSW
Hemsley House
20 Roslyn Street
Potts Point
NSW 2011
Ph: 02 9356 0450
Fax: 02 9357 2334

Endometriosis Association VIC
37 Andrew Crescent
South Croydon
VIC 3136

Endometriosis Support Group QLD
Penny Fenton
Ph: 07 5521 0507

Women's Health Victoria

Ph: 03 9662 3755
Health Information Line:
Ph: 03 9662 3742
Email: whv@whv.org.au
Website: www.whv.org.au

New Zealand
New Zealand Endometriosis Association

PO Box 1683
Palmerston North
Ph/fax: 06 359 2613
Email: nzendo@xtra.co.nz
Website: www.nzendo.co.nz

United Kingdom
Endometriosis Society

Helpline: 020 7222 2776

National Association for Premenstrual Syndrome

7 Swifts Court
High Street
Seal
Kent TN15 OEG

Postal: PO Box 72,
Sevenoaks,Kent TN15 OEG
Ph/fax: 0173 276 0011
Helpline: 0173 276 0012
Email: naps@charity.vfree.com
Website: www.pms.org.uk

Women's Health

A Resource, information and
support centre.
52 Featherstone Street
London EC1Y 8RT
Ph: 020 7251 6580
Website:
www.womenshealthlondon.org.uk

MORE WEBSITES

These websites are also worth
checking out, and will link you to
more:
www.menstruation.com
www.endometriosisassn.org
www.yoni.com

References

Amann-Gainotti M. 'Sexual socialisation during early adolescence: the menarche.' *Adolescence* 1986 Fall; 21(83):703-10

Amann-Gainotti M. 'Knowledge and beliefs about the body interior during early adolescence: the case of menstruations.' *Acta Paedopsychiatry* 1989; 52(2):143-9

Brown W, Fernandez E. 'Relationships between pain and mood state during the menstrual cycle.' In: Kenny DT and Job RFS, editors. *Australia's Adolescents* University of New England Press; Armidale. 1995; 257-261.

Campbell BC, Udry JR. 'Stress and age at menarche of mothers and daughters.' *Journal of Biosociological Science* 1995 Apr;27(2):127-34

Delaney Janice, Mary Jane Lupton and Emily Toth *The Curse: A Cultural History of Menstruation* University of Illinois Press: Chicago 1988

Diamant Anita *The Red Tent* Allen and Unwin: St Leonards, NSW 1998

Elium Jeanne and Don *Raising A Daughter* Celestial Arts: Berkeley 1994

Friday Nancy *My Mother/My Self* Fontana Collins: London 1981

Gillooly Jessica B. *Before She Gets Her Period* Perspective Publishing: Los Angeles 1998

Grahn Judy *Blood, Bread and Roses* Beacon Press: Boston 1993

Koff E, Rierdan J. 'Premenarcheal expectations and postmenarcheal experiences of positive and negative menstrual related changes.' *Journal of Adolescent Health* 1996 Apr;18(4):286-91

Mahr E. 'Perception of the First Menstruation.' *Geburshilfe Fraeenheilkd* 1987 Nov; 47(11):812-6

McGrory A. 'Menarche: responses of early adolescent females.' *Adolescence* 1990 Summer; 25(98):265-70

Owen Lara *Her Blood is Gold* Aquarian/Thorsons: London 1993

Patton GC, Hibbert ME, Cartlin J et al. 'Menarche and the onset of depression and anxiety in Victoria, Australia.' *Journal of Epidemiology and Community Health* 1996 Dec; 50(6):661-6

Pillemer DB, Koff E, Rhinehart ED, Rierdan J. 'Flashbulb memories of menarche and adult menstrual distress.' *Journal of Adolescence* 1987 Jun; 10(2):187-99

Teperi J, Rimpela M. 'Menstrual pain, health and behavior in girls.' *Social Science Medicine* 1989; 29(2): 163-9

PART 1: OUR CYCLING BODIES

Amann-Gainotti M. 'Knowledge and beliefs about the body interior during early adolescence: the case of menstruations.' *Acta Paedopsychiatry* 1989; 52(2):143-9

Angier Natalie *Woman: An Intimate Geography* Virago Press: London 1999

Australian Bureau of Statistics *2001 Year Book* Australia McCarron, Bird and Co. Melbourne 2001

Brown W, Fernandez E. 'Relationships between pain and mood state during the menstrual cycle.' In: Kenny DT and Job RFS, editors. *Australia's Adolescents* University of New England Press; Armidale. 1995; 257-261.

Campbell BC, Udry JR. 'Stress and age at menarche of mothers and daughters.' *Journal of Biosociological Science* 1995 Apr; 27(2):127-34

Frank Otto and Mirjam Pressler (eds)*The Definitive Edition: The Diary of a Young Girl: Anne Frank* Bantam Books: New York 1991

Gillooly Jessica B. *Before She Gets Her Period* Perspective Publishing: Los Angeles 1998

Koff E, Rierdan J. 'Premenarcheal expectations and postmenarcheal experiences of positive and negative menstrual related changes.' *Journal of Adolescent Health* 1996 Apr;18(4):286-91

Llewellyn-Jones Derek and Suzanne Abraham *Everygirl* Oxford University Press: Oxford 1986,1989

Maciocia Giovanni *Obstetrics and Gynecology in Chinese Medicine* Churchill Livingstone: New York 1998

Mahr E. 'Perception of the First Menstruation.' *Geburshilfe Fraeenheilkd* 1987 Nov; 47(11):812-6

McGrory A. 'Menarche: responses of early adolescent females.' *Adolescence* 1990 Summer; 25(98):265-70

Montero P, Bernis C, Fernandez V, Castro S. 'Influence of body mass index and slimming habits on menstrual pain and cycle irregularity.' *Journal of Biosocial Science* 1996 Jul; 28(3):315-23

Naish Francesca *The Lunar Cycle* Nature and Health Books: Australia 1989

Naish Francesca *Natural Fertility* Sally Milner Publishing: Bowral 1993, 2001

Northrup Christiane *Women's Bodies, Women's Wisdom* Bantam Books: New York 1994

Pillemer DB, Koff E, Rhinehart ED, Rierdan J. 'Flashbulb memories of menarche and adult menstrual distress.' *Journal of Adolescence* 1987 Jun; 10(2):187-99

Sanders JL. 'Relation of personal space to the human menstrual cycle.' *Journal of Psychology* 1978 Nov;100(2nd Half):275-8

Trickey Ruth *Women, Hormones and The Menstrual Cycle* Allen and Unwin: Sydney 1998

Trickey Ruth and Kaz Cooke *Women's Troubles* Allen and Unwin: Sydney 1998

Van De Graaff Kent M. and Fox Stuart Ira *Concepts of Hunam Anatomy and Physiology* (Second Edition) Wm C. Brown Publishers: Dubuque Iowa 1989

PART 2: BLESSING OR CURSE

Angier Natalie *Woman: An Intimate Geography* Virago Press: London 1999

Baker Jeannine and Frederick, and Tamara Slayton *Conscious Conception* Freestone Publishing: Monroe, Utah 1986

Blaffer Hrdy Sarah *Mother Nature* Chatto & Windus: London 1999

Bolen Jean Shinoda *Goddesses in Every Woman* Harper and Row: New York 1985

Broom D. 'Gendering health, sexing illness' *Proceedings of the Third National Women's Health Conference*: Australia 1995.

Coutinho Elsimar M. *Is Menstruation Obsolete?* Oxford University Press: New York 1999

Delaney Janice, Mary Jane Lupton and Emily Toth *The Curse: A Cultural History of Menstruation* University of Illinois Press: Chicago 1988

De Rovere Tiziana *Sacred Fire* Celestial Arts: Berkeley 1995

Diamant Anita *The Red Tent* Allen and Unwin: St Leonards, NSW 1998

Estes Clarissa Pinkola *Women Who Run With Wolve*s Rider: London 1992

Grahn Judy *Blood, Bread and Roses* Beacon Press: Boston 1993

Grant Ellen *The Bitter Pill* Elm Tree Books: London 1985

Greer Germaine *The Female Eunuch* McGraw-Hill: New York 1971

Hall Calvin S. and Vernon J. Nordby *A Primer of Jungian Psychology* Meridian: New York 1973

Hulley Charles E. *Dreamtime Moon* Reed Books: Sydney 1996

Iyengar Geeta S. *Yoga A Gem for Women* Allied Publishers Private Limited: New Delhi 1983

Jung C.G. *The Practice of Psychotherapy* Princeton University Press: New York 1954

Little William et al. *The Shorter Oxford English Dictionary* Clarendon Press: Oxford 1964

MacKenzie Vicki Tenzin Palmo: *Cave in the Snow* 1998

McCauley Lucy, Carlson Amy G, and Leo Jennifer (eds) *A Woman's Path* Travelers' Tales Books: San Francisco 2000

McLynn Frank *A Biography: Carl Gustav Jung* Transworld: London 1996

Naish Francesca *The Lunar Cycle* Nature and Health Books: Australia 1989

Naish Francesca *Natural Fertility* Sally Milner Publishing: Bowral 1993, 2001

Northrup Christiane *Women's Bodies, Women's Wisdom* Bantam Books: New York 1994

McTaggart Lynne *What Doctors Don't Tell You* Thorsons: London 1996

Owen Lara *Her Blood is Gold* Aquarian/Thorsons: London 1993

Seaman Barbara *The Doctors Case Against the Pill* Hunter House: Alameda, California 1969, 1995

Shuttle Penelope and Peter Redgrove *The Wise Wound* Paladin Grafton Books: London 1978

Tarnas Richard *The Passion of the Western Mind* Ballantine Books: New York 1991

Tavris Carol *Mismeasure of Woman* Simon and Schuster: New York 1992

Weideger Paula *Female Cycles* The Women's Press: London 1975

White David Gordon *The Alchemical Body* University of Chicago Press: Chicago 1996

Widdows Richard ed. 'The coming of age' *Family of Man* Part 5 Marshall Cavendish: Great Britain 1974

PART 3: RITE OF PASSAGE

Amann-Gainotti M. 'Knowledge and beliefs about the body interior during early adolescence: the case of menstruations.' *Acta Paedopsychiatry* 1989; 52(2):143-9

Brown W, Fernandez E. 'Relationships between pain and mood state during the menstrual cycle.' In: Kenny DT and Job RFS, editors.

Australia's Adolescents University of New England Press; Armidale. 1995; 257-261.

Campbell BC, Udry JR. 'Stress and age at menarche of mothers and daughters.' *Journal of Biosociological Science* 1995 Apr; 27(2):127-34

Carr-Nangle RE, Johnson WG, Bergeron KC, Nangle DW. 'Body image changes over the menstrual cycle in normal women.' *International Journal of Eating Disorders* 1994 Nov; 16(3):267-73

Costello A, Vallely B and Young J. *The Sanitary Protection Scandal* Aldgate Press: London 1989

Delaney Janice, Mary Jane Lupton and Emily Toth *The Curse: A Cultural History of Menstruation* University of Illinois Press: Chicago 1988

De Rovere Tiziana *Sacred Fire* Celestial Arts: Berkeley 1995

Diamant Anita *The Red Tent* Allen and Unwin: St Leonards, NSW 1998

Elium Jeanne and Don *Raising A Daughter* Celestial Arts: Berkeley 1994

Fredriksson Marianne *Hanna's Daughters* Phoenix Books: London 1994

Friday Nancy *My Mother/My Self* Fontana Collins: London 1981

Gillooly Jessica B. *Before She Gets Her Period* Perspective Publishing: Los Angeles 1998

Grahn Judy *Blood, Bread and Roses* Beacon Press: Boston 1993

Gravelle Karen and Jennifer *The Period Book* Walker and Company: New York 1996

Koff E, Rierdan J. 'Premenarcheal expectations and postmenarcheal experiences of positive and negative menstrual related changes.' *Journal of Adolescent Health* 1996 Apr;18(4):286-91

Llewellyn-Jones Derek and Suzanne Abraham *Everygirl* Oxford University Press: Oxford 1986,1989

Mahr E. 'Perception of the First Menstruation.' *Geburshilfe Fraeenheilkd* 1987 Nov;47(11):812-6

McGrory A. 'Menarche: responses of early adolescent females.' *Adolescence* 1990 Summer; 25(98):265-70

Northrup Christiane *Women's Bodies, Women's Wisdom* Bantam Books: New York 1994

O'Grady Kathleen and Paula Wansbrough *Sweet Secrets* Second Story Press: Toronto 1997

Owen Lara *Her Blood is Gold* Aquarian/Thorsons: London 1993

Patton GC, Hibbert ME, Cartlin J et al. 'Menarche and the onset of depression and anxiety in Victoria, Australia.' *Journal of Epidemiology and Community Health* 1996 Dec; 50(6):661-6

Pillemer DB, Koff E, Rhinehart ED, Rierdan J. 'Flashbulb memories of menarche and adult menstrual distress.' *Journal of Adolescence* 1987 Jun; 10(2):187-99

Pipher Mary *Reviving Ophelia* Doubleday: Australia 1996

Rutter Virginia Beane *Celebrating Girls* MJF Books: New York 1996

Teperi J, Rimpela M. 'Menstrual pain, health and behavior in girls.' *Social Science Medicine* 1989; 29(2): 163-9

Widdows Richard ed. 'The coming of age' *Family of Man* Part 5 Marshall Cavendish: Great Britain 1974

PART 4: PROBLEM PERIODS

Amann-Gainotti M. 'Sexual socialisation during early adolescence: the menarche.' *Adolescence* 1986 Fall;21(83):703-10

Amann-Gainotti M. 'Knowledge and beliefs about the body interior during early adolescence: the case of menstruations.' *Acta Paedopsychiatry* 1989; 52(2):143-9

Angier Natalie *Woman: An Intimate Geography* Virago Press: London 1999

Armstrong June and Bruce Sutherland *Menstrual Wellness* Collins Dove: Melbourne 1987

Australian Bureau of Statistics *2001 Year Book Australia* McCarron, Bird and Co. Melbourne 2001

Baker Jeannine and Frederick, and Tamara Slayton *Conscious Conception* Freestone Publishing: Monroe, Utah 1986

Blaffer Hrdy Sarah *Mother Nature* Chatto & Windus: London 1999

Bodley Lisa *Recreating Menstruation* Gnana Yoga Foundation: Melbourne 1995

Bolen Jean Shinoda *Goddesses in Every Woman* Harper and Row: New York 1985

Broom D. 'Gendering health, sexing illness' *Proceedings of the Third National Women's Health Conference*: Australia 1995.

Brown W, Fernandez E. 'Relationships between pain and mood state during the menstrual cycle.' In: Kenny DT and Job RFS, editors. *Australia's Adolescents* University of New England Press; Armidale. 1995; 257-261.

Campbell BC, Udry JR. 'Stress and age at menarche of mothers and daughters.' *Journal of Biosociological Science* 1995 Apr;27(2):127-34

Carr-Nangle RE, Johnson WG, Bergeron KC, Nangle DW. 'Body image changes over the menstrual cycle in normal women.' *International Journal of Eating Disorders* 1994 Nov;16(3):267-73

Donohoe Mark Dr 'Human rusting — startling new discoveries about iron.' *Natural Health* 1993 Aug/Sept; Vol 6, No.5: 2-3

Grant Ellen *The Bitter Pill* Elm Tree Books: London 1985

Gravelle Karen and Jennifer *The Period Book* Walker and Company: New York 1996

Llewellyn-Jones Derek and Suzanne Abraham *Everygirl* Oxford University Press: Oxford 1986,1989

Lonsdorf Nancy, Veronica Butler and Melanie Brown *A Woman's Best Medicine* Putnam: New York 1995

Maciocia Giovanni *Obstetrics and Gynecology in Chinese Medicine* Churchill Livingstone: New York 1998

Montero P, Bernis C, Fernandez V, Castro S. 'Influence of body mass index and slimming habits on menstrual pain and cycle irregularity.' *Journal of Biosocial Science* 1996 Jul;28(3):315-23

Morrison Judith H. *The Book of Ayurveda* Simon and Schuster: Sydney 1994

Naish Francesca *The Lunar Cycle* Nature and Health Books: Australia 1989

Naish Francesca *Natural Fertility* Sally Milner Publishing: Bowral 1993, 2001

Northrup Christiane *Women's Bodies, Women's Wisdom* Bantam Books: New York 1994

McTaggart Lynne *What Doctors Don't Tell You* Thorsons: London 1996

Patton GC, Hibbert ME, Cartlin J et al. 'Menarche and the onset of depression and anxiety in Victoria, Australia.' *Journal of Epidemiology and Community Health* 1996 Dec; 50(6):661-6

Pillemer DB, Koff E, Rhinehart ED, Rierdan J. 'Flashbulb memories of menarche and adult menstrual distress.' *Journal of Adolescence* 1987 Jun; 10(2):187-99

Roberts J. (ed.) 'The Pill and sex — risks to health and fertility' *The Foresight Association Newsletter*: Australia 1995

Seaman Barbara *The Doctors Case Against the Pill* Hunter House: Alameda, California 1969,1995

Scott Julian and Susan *Natural Medicine for Women* Simon and Schuster: Sydney 1988

Trickey Ruth *Women, Hormones and The Menstrual Cycle* Allen and Unwin: Sydney 1998

Trickey Ruth and Kaz Cooke *Women's Troubles* Allen and Unwin: Sydney 1998

Yu Jin M.D. *Handbook of Obstetrics and Gynecology in Chinese Medicine* Eastland Press: Seattle 1998

PART 5: LEARNING TO RIDE THE MENSTRUAL CYCLE

Colborn Theo, John Peterson Myers and Dianne Dumanoski *Our Stolen Future* Little, Brown and Company: Boston 1996

Friday Nancy *My Mother/My Self* Fontana Collins: London 1981

Howard Judy *Bach Flower Remedies for Women* The C.W.Daniel Company: London 1992

Iyengar Geeta S. *Yoga A Gem for Women* Allied Publishers Private Limited: New Delhi 1983

Lonsdorf Nancy, Veronica Butler and Melanie Brown *A Woman's Best Medicine* Putnam: New York 1995

Maciocia Giovanni *Obstetrics and Gynecology in Chinese Medicine* Churchill Livingstone: New York 1998

Montero P, Bernis C, Fernandez V, Castro S. 'Influence of body mass index and slimming habits on menstrual pain and cycle irregularity.' *Journal of Biosocial Science* 1996 Jul;28(3):315-23

Morrison Judith H. *The Book of Ayurveda* Simon and Schuster: Sydney 1994

Naish Francesca *The Lunar Cycle* Nature and Health Books: Australia 1989

Naish Francesca *Natural Fertility* Sally Milner Publishing: Bowral 1993, 2001

Northrup Christiane *Women's Bodies, Women's Wisdom* Bantam Books: New York 1994

Patton GC, Hibbert ME, Cartlin J et al. 'Menarche and the onset of depression and anxiety in Victoria, Australia.' *Journal of Epidemiology and Community Health* 1996 Dec; 50(6):661-6

Pillemer DB, Koff E, Rhinehart ED, Rierdan J. 'Flashbulb memories of menarche and adult menstrual distress.' *Journal of Adolescence* 1987 Jun; 10(2):187-99

Pope Alexandra *The Wild Genie* Sally Milner Publishing: Bowral, Australia 2001

Scott Julian and Susan *Natural Medicine for Women* Simon and Schuster: Sydney 1988

Tavris Carol *Mismeasure of Woman* Simon and Schuster: New York 1992

Teperi J, Rimpela M. 'Menstrual pain, health and behavior in girls.' *Social Science Medicine* 1989; 29(2): 163-9

Trickey Ruth Women, *Hormones and The Menstrual Cycle* Allen and Unwin: Sydney 1998

Trickey Ruth and Kaz Cooke *Women's Troubles* Allen and Unwin: Sydney 1998

THE BLESSING

Day Marele *The Lambs of God* Allen and Unwin: Sydney 1997

Recommended reading

A Woman's Best Medicine Nancy Lonsdorf, Veronica Butler and
Melanie Brown
Putnam: New York 1995
**An inspiring and thorough introduction to Ayur-veda, especially as it
relates to women's health.**

Before She Gets Her Period Jessica Gillooly
Perspective Publishing, 1998
**A friendly book using personal stories, exercises and activities to help
parents talk with their daughters about menstruation — even if their
daughters don't want to talk.**

Blood, Bread and Roses Judy Grahn
Beacon Press: Boston 1993
**A very interesting exploration into the historic importance of
menstruation, it's influence on mathematics, culture and our concepts
of time.**

Her Blood is Gold Lara Owen
The Aquarian Press, London 1993
**A truly wonderful book. Well written, positive and affirming. Drawing
on myth, tradition, and personal stories which turn pain,
embarrassment, and self-consciousness about menstruation into
creativity, self-fulfilment, and healing.**

Menstruation Resource Kit
  Moontime Menstrual Traders, PO Box 836, Whakatu/Nelson,
  Aotearoa/New Zealand
**Information on: Supporting Our Daughters, Menstruation and our
World, Menstrual Products — the Options, The Menstrual Cycle —
Cycling On, Pre menstrual Syndrome — Pre Menstrual Strength,
Menopause — Growing Wise, Menstrual Health — Feeling Good
Well put together, accessible and beautifully presented.**

Natural Fertility Francesca Naish
  Sally Milner Publishing, Sydney 1991
**A 'must have' book about empowerment through awareness of our
cycles and fertile times, information which can then be used for
contraception and conception, as well as indicators of hormonal
health. Comprehensive sections on the physiology of the menstrual
cycle, problems with unnatural forms of contraception, natural
remedies for hormonal health and much more. Useful for women
from menarche to menopause.**

Recreating Menstruation Lisa Bodley
  Gnana Yoga Foundation, Melbourne 1995
**A very clear and deceptively simple book about the Taoist 'Deer
Exercise' for women. An excellent daily practice useful for menstrual
problems and hormonal imbalance.**

Sweet Secrets Kathleen O'Grady and Paula Wansbrough
  Second Story Press: Toronto 1997
**Positive and inspiring personal and cultural stories of menarche and
menstruation.**

The Period Book Karen and Jennifer Gravelle
  Walker and Company: New York 1996
**Written by a teenage girl and her aunt this book for girls is
informative and approachable.**

The Red Tent Anita Diamant
   Allen and Unwin: St Leonards, NSW 1998
Based on the story of Rachel from the Old Testament, this a beautifully told story of the menstrual rituals of the red tent. Inspiring and fascinating.

The Wild Genie Alexandra Pope
   Sally Milner Publishing: Bowral 2001
A beautifully written book by psychotherapist, Alexandra Pope, exploring women's painful and difficult menstrual experiences. Lots of well-grounded practical information as well as thought provoking stories and understandings about the subtleties of the menstrual experience.

The Wise Wound Penelope Shuttle & Peter Redgrove
   Paladin Grafton Books, London 1986
Also a great book. Explores the historical and cultural legacy of menstrual repression. A fascinating reinterpretation of the central myths of Christianity, witch trials, vampire movies and more.

Woman: An Intimate Geography Natalie Angier
   Virago Press: London 1999
Well researched and very readable Natalie Angier explores and interprets the most up to date research on women's physiology.

Women, Hormones and The Menstrual Cycle Ruth Trickey
   Allen and Unwin: Sydney 1998
A very thorough book written by herbalist Ruth Trickey. A good one for your book shelf.

Women's Bodies, Women's Wisdom Christiane Northrup, M.D.
   Bantam Books, New York 1994, revised 1998
A well considered book. A good combination of medical know how from an obstetrician/gynaecologist who has a holistic approach and great appreciation for the body-mind connection.

Women's Trouble Ruth Trickey & Kaz Cooke
  Allen & Unwin, Sydney 1998

A very approachable book covering many topics of interest from feral hormones to surgery to anatomy combining the humour of Kaz Cooke and expertise of Ruth Trickey. Fun to read and teenage friendly. (See also Real Gorgeous by Kaz Cooke. No-nonsense information about size, shape, self esteem and the cellulite scam. It will make you laugh and help you make friends with your body.)

About the author

With a background in social work and hypnotherapy, Jane Bennett is Australia's National Coordinator of Natural Fertility Management. She is particularly interested in transforming inherited views of embarrassment and shame around menstruation to a positive and empowering experience, and helping women tune into the cycles of nature through their own menstrual cycles. Herself a mother and daughter, she is passionate about working with girls and young women and since 2000 has been running A Blessing Not a Curse workshops for mothers and daughters.